WHEN SOMEONE YOU LOVE IS BIPOLAR

When Someone You Love Is Bipolar

Help and Support for You and Your Partner

Cynthia G. Last, PhD

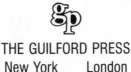

THE GUILFORD PRESS
New York   London

Library of Congress Cataloging-in-Publication Data

Last, Cynthia G.
    When someone you love is bipolar : help and support for you and
your partner / Cynthia G. Last.
        p.   cm.
    Includes index.
    ISBN 978-1-60623-124-1 (hardcover : alk. paper)
    ISBN 978-1-59385-608-3 (pbk. : alk. paper)
    1. Manic–depressive illness—Popular works.   2. Families of the
mentally ill.   I. Title.
    RC516.L37 2009
    616.89′5—dc22

                                                2008048492

Contents

Foreword   vii

Acknowledgments   xi

Introduction   1

1 Does Someone You Love Have Bipolar Disorder?   7

2 What You Can Expect: 31
   The Course of Bipolar Illness

3 "It's Not Me!": When Your Partner Is in Denial   61

4 What You Need to Know about Your   86
   Partner's Treatment

5 You, Your Loved One, and the Doctors: 125
   The Team Approach to Getting and Staying Well

6 Helping Your Partner Stick with Medication   145

7 Other Things You and Your Partner Can Do   165
   to Prevent Mood Episodes

8 Strategies for Dealing with the Ups Together   199

9 Strategies for Dealing with the Downs Together   235

10 Taking Care of Yourself and Your Relationship   260

Resources   283

Index   293

About the Author   306

Foreword

It was a Friday night in early spring and I had just returned from a long business trip. Out for a quiet, relaxing dinner with friends, I glanced around the restaurant and caught sight of her. A mutual friend introduced us, and, as they say, that was the beginning.

I waited a couple of days and then called Cynthia. Our first date was magical, and as it drew to a close we made plans for the next night. From that point on we were together almost every night. We grew very close in a short period of time, and soon my feelings turned into love and I knew that I wanted to spend the rest of my life with this incredible woman. She was everything I had ever hoped for in a mate—beautiful, intelligent, affectionate, spontaneous, exuberant, bursting with passion and enthusiasm for life. I felt very fortunate indeed.

But during the early years of our marriage Cynthia's mood would, at times, shift rapidly, seemingly for no reason. It was hard to understand. In a matter of minutes she would go from warm and bubbly to angry and argumentative, and then hours later she would be back to her normal self. There also were the occasional down periods that came on more gradually and lasted for days at a time. Sometimes I thought Cynthia was just being difficult, spoiled, or self-centered. Other times I worried that perhaps her feelings for me had changed.

But as the mood swings became more frequent and intense, it became clear that something was terribly wrong. I remember one of those awful days when my wife, tears streaming down her face, pleaded with me to "*Please* take it away," telling me emphatically, "I don't want to be this way!" My heart still breaks every time I recall the helpless look on her face. It was then that I realized how much Cynthia was suffering and that we had to get help.

Although we sought professional help, and the doctors put forth their best efforts, it took quite a while for their hard work to pay off. Part of this was due to my wife's reluctance to accept that she had bipolar disorder. To be honest, I had trouble accepting it too. I think it was because the version of bipolar disorder that Cynthia has—a relatively mild type, known as type II—doesn't appear the way the illness is portrayed in movies and on TV, with full-blown out-of-control behavior. Instead, it includes a less severe form of mania known as *hypo*mania that sometimes is subtle and hard for even experienced mental health professionals to pinpoint.

But as the evidence in favor of the type II bipolar diagnosis mounted, Cynthia eventually came to accept it, and so did I. In a way I was relieved. It meant my wife's feelings for me hadn't changed, that it wasn't our relationship that was the problem. It was *an illness* that was causing her to act the way she did.

Unfortunately, after we both accepted the diagnosis, we still had more obstacles ahead. Cynthia didn't have a positive response to most of the drugs typically used to treat bipolar disorder, so it took several doctors, trials of numerous medications, and many years to get the right medications in place. The fact that we did get there, to a regimen that has kept Cynthia on an even keel for years, was also due in part to both of our efforts. At my suggestion, because I understood my wife's high regard for quantifying problems, Cynthia religiously charted her daily drug dosages and moods to figure out which medications were working. And although it wasn't always easy to be optimistic in the face of the many disappointments we experienced, I never gave up hope that we would find an effective treatment and continued to encourage my wife. Ultimately we had the satisfaction of knowing that together we had made our own contribution to finding the treatment that has done Cynthia so much good.

But it wasn't only the medication that helped stabilize Cynthia's mood. My wife and I have taken other steps together as a couple too. One really beneficial discovery was how critical it is to avoid or minimize, whenever possible, situations, events, or circumstances that are likely to cause mood problems. Knowing my wife as well as I do, because of the ongoing open and honest communication we have, I'm aware of Cynthia's triggers and am able to navigate her away from them—just like someone would steer a person walking on crutches away from cracks in the sidewalk. I do this now without even thinking because it has become part of our routine.

I'm not suggesting that I haven't made sacrifices to help my wife manage her illness. They are, however, minor, and most of them have involved making lifestyle changes. For example, as you'll learn in this book, following a set routine is very important to mood stability, which means travel is often a problem for people with bipolar disorder. So Cynthia and I don't take trips that involve extensive travel as much as I'd like. Instead, we frequently take "day trips" to places we haven't been before; that way our sense of adventure doesn't go entirely unfulfilled.

We also don't stay at parties as late as I want to. We don't decline invitations; we just leave an hour or two before we might have in the past, because Cynthia and I know that a consistent sleep schedule is so vital to mood stability. Small modifications like this often produce such large gains that it's difficult to believe they ever seemed like hardships at all.

During the years that Cynthia was having frequent mood episodes, we had "spotty" social lives. Consequently, there were few people I could turn to when I felt alone. But to tell you the truth, I found the best coping strategy for me actually wasn't to talk to other people. It was to devote time to my hobbies and interests, which allowed me to take a mental break. Everyone has to find a way to let off steam and refuel in the face of a challenge like bipolar disorder. I found mine in the activities I had always found rejuvenating, and they retained their positive power for me in part because my wife never failed to remind me how important it was that I preserve that part of my life. So I did and still do.

In turn, I encourage and support Cynthia's dedication to her work. Cynthia's professional life—her practice as a clinical psychologist, her research, her writing—has always been a source of fulfillment and joy for her. And to her good fortune, her career has flourished over the years despite her illness. For example, even in the depth of a severe depression many years ago, Cynthia wrote what turned out to be an award-winning research grant. I think, in a way, that her work at times provided her an escape from herself, much in the same way that my hobbies generated a distraction for me. Knowing this, we unfailingly support each other's efforts to pursue personal and professional growth and fulfillment. Bipolar disorder is a fact of our life together, but it has never been our *whole* life together. We lead separate lives as individuals with our own interests and goals, and we protect our life as a couple as well.

I firmly believe that my wife's having bipolar illness has made us much closer and stronger as a couple because of how we have had to come together to fight this dragon. We are very appreciative of the good times and of each other—we virtually never take each other for granted. I also believe that I'm a better person because of having to help my wife with this illness. I've learned to listen, to be compassionate, and to give of myself from the heart, without necessarily expecting anything in return.

Cynthia and I have been together now for 22 years and celebrated our 20th wedding anniversary last fall. Although each of us received several gifts on that special day, the best gift of all was the one we had created together. With a lot of love and hard work, the two of us have been able to achieve a stable and wonderful life. We've refused to let bipolar disorder take over our relationship.

My wife has written this book so that you and your partner can benefit from all that we've learned. If only we had had a book like this to help guide us along the way, I know both of us would have suffered much less.

As they say, although life and love are never easy, it's the reward that makes the effort worthwhile. Put in the effort and reap the reward of a stable and wonderful life. We've done it, many of Cynthia's patients and their partners have done it, and, I expect, you and your loved one can do it too.

With my best wishes for you and your family,

BARRY M. RUBIN

Acknowledgments

Good ideas can come at the most unexpected times. The idea for this book arose during a power outage following a severe hurricane. With little to do for entertainment—no computer or TV, and shops, movie theaters, and restaurants all closed—I put pen to paper and sketched out a rough outline for a book on bipolar disorder. In it I envisioned using my dual perspective on the illness, gleaned from both my personal and professional experiences.

The decision to "come out of the closet"—to reveal that I have bipolar disorder (albeit a mild version)—did not, as you might imagine, come easily. I pondered at some length the potential consequences of taking this action, and there was one individual in particular who helped me through this process, my colleague Lori Grabois, MD. For her insight and candor, I owe Lori my deepest gratitude.

There are other people who helped in various ways during the writing of this book. Special thanks are due my friend and colleague Ana Kelton-Brand, PhD, for allowing me to use her as a sounding board when I needed someone to talk to about some of the book's topics. My appreciation goes to Priti Kothari, MD, for reviewing the material in Chapter 4 on medical treatments. My love and thanks go to my husband, Barry Rubin, for the many roles he played in bringing this book to fruition—commenting on some of the book's material, writing the foreword, and supporting me throughout. My respect and heartfelt thanks go to my two wonderful editors at The Guilford Press, Kitty

Moore and Christine Benton, who helped me, each in her own talented way, produce the very best work I was capable of.

I also want to take this opportunity to acknowledge the remarkable group of professionals that I had the good fortune to have as mentors earlier in my career. These individuals—David H. Barlow, PhD, Michel Hersen, PhD, David J. Kupfer, MD, and the late Joaquim Puig-Antich, MD—played pivotal roles in shaping my professional development, including how I approach clinical problems.

My thanks also go to members of my family, especially my father, Morton Last, my mother, Sally Mailman, and my sister, Maxine Last, for seeing me through my many moods over the years. No matter what, they were always there.

Finally, I always will be most appreciative of the patients and partners I've had the privilege to work with. It is from them—their triumphs and defeats—that we can learn so much, and then go on to enrich others' lives.

WHEN SOMEONE YOU LOVE IS BIPOLAR

Introduction

Kevin describes Ashley's life as like a roller coaster ride. Sometimes she's really "up" and excited—bursting with energy, filled with enthusiasm, and feeling like she's on top of the world. Other times it's the exact opposite: her mood is way down, she's lethargic, and she's negative about everything, including being certain her misery never will end.

When Ashley's feeling good she acts impulsively—speeds, goes on spending sprees, drinks too much—and doesn't think of the potential negative consequences of her actions. Kevin has tried to caution her when she's like this, but Ashley gets angry and accuses him of being "a stick in the mud." So during these periods he's learned it's best to keep silent but stay "on alert," like a firefighter waiting for the next emergency call.

When Ashley's depressed there are problems too. She has trouble at her job—missing days, not getting her work done, and isolating herself from her coworkers by keeping her office door shut. She worries about losing her job, and though Kevin tries to reassure her, the truth is he's worried too. Could they manage without his wife's income? Would she be okay if she were home all day instead of away and occupied, or would she get even more depressed?

Ashley has bipolar disorder, also known as manic–depressive illness. And although Kevin's moods are no different from the average person's ups and downs, he's carried along on the roller coaster ride with

1

his wife. Her unpredictable mood swings are extremely difficult for Kevin to live with, as is the fallout that follows her highs and lows. Whether it's meeting expectations at work, keeping up with friends and family, pursuing hobbies and interests, and, at times, even just taking care of the basics of sleeping, eating, and grooming—bipolar disorder makes day-to-day life a challenge for both of them.

If your spouse or partner has this illness, he or she is hardly alone, nor are you. In fact, bipolar disorder is present in more than 3% of our population. Although it occurs in children and adolescents, the disorder appears most frequently in adults. It's equally common in men and women and cuts across all races, ethnic and cultural backgrounds, religions, and economic levels. And it occurs across the globe.

Some of the greatest minds and talents of our times have had bipolar disorder, including world-renowned politicians, artists, actors, musicians, and writers. Winston Churchill, Ernest Hemingway, Vincent van Gogh, and Robert Schumann are just a few of the remarkable individuals who have suffered from this disorder. Most of the people who have this problem, however, would not necessarily be considered extraordinary. Like Ashley, and probably like the person you care so much about, they're regular people who just want to lead normal lives.

I know about the goals and aspirations of bipolar people because of my professional and personal experience with the illness. Being a clinical psychologist, I have treated bipolar individuals and their families for more than a quarter of a century. But as or more important, although fortunate to have a relatively mild version of the condition, I have bipolar disorder myself.

I ignored the obvious for as long as I possibly could. I say "ignored the obvious" because, as I said, having diagnosed and treated bipolar disorder in my practice I was well aware of how the illness manifests itself. This knowledge, however, didn't help me accept what was there to see, that my problem wasn't "personality quirks" or depression. Although, in retrospect, it's clear that I had had bipolar disorder since adolescence, it wasn't until my 30s that I got the correct diagnosis, and it wasn't until I turned 40 that I believed it was true.

Because I've had this disorder most of my life and because I've treated so many bipolar individuals and their families, I know the effects this illness has not just on the person who has the disorder but also on the people who are close by, especially spouses and partners.

In my situation I have seen how much my husband of 20 years has been affected by my illness, watching him suffer along with me during my mood episodes, day after day, week after week, feeling helpless to change my course. Thank goodness once I finally accepted the diagnosis I was able to get the right treatment—the correct medication and self-help strategies—to keep the pendulum from swinging too far in one direction or the other. So now both my husband and I are leading stable lives.

Helplessness is only one of the feelings that spouses and partners of people with bipolar disorder experience. Fear and worry also are common emotions. It can be very scary—for those of you who have loved ones who have the more severe form of the illness—to watch the out-of-control behavior that can occur during manic highs and to live through the horrendous aftermath of serious risk-taking behavior. It also can be frightening to watch your spouse or partner during the low times, when he or she is unable or barely able to follow a normal routine or gets so despondent that death seems like the only answer.

Watching someone you love go through mood swings can be heartbreaking. If you are an especially sensitive and empathetic person, you may actually feel the emotional pain that your loved one is experiencing, and possibly even have mood problems yourself (not of the same magnitude as those with bipolar disorder, but real and painful nonetheless) as a result of living with someone with this illness.

On the other hand you may be angry—angry at how your partner's mood swings are affecting you and, if you have children, the rest of your family. Kevin feels this way. His family is struggling with the financial consequences of Ashley's bipolar disorder—because of lost work time and excessive spending—as well as the effects the illness has had on their two young children, whose care often falls to Kevin, particularly when Ashley has been drinking or is depressed. The relationship between Ashley and her husband is, to say the least, strained, as are the couple's relationships with friends and relatives: Ashley keeps to herself at home when she's depressed, just as she does at her workplace. Because of all this, Kevin, understandably, is irritable and short-tempered.

Kevin and Ashley are concerned about the future for another reason: bipolar illness is a largely genetic disorder. If you too have children, you may be worried that one of your offspring will end up with the disorder, and if you see early warning signs of the illness in your child you may feel that you are to blame and terribly guilty. If you are in this situation, please know that in the 21st century we are at a time of great advances in the treatment of bipolar disorder, in both pharmacological and psychological therapies, so you don't need to be so afraid for your child—or your mate either for that matter—or filled with guilt.

Feelings of shame and secrecy also may be part of the bipolar experience for you and your loved one. Trying to keep the mood swings "quiet" and away from other people—friends, employers, employees, even relatives—can be an enormous, exhausting task. If mood swings can't be kept private, because of manic behavior that occurs outside the home or depressed behavior that keeps your partner from being able to meet responsibilities, like going to work, you may feel embarrassed or ashamed.

You may often feel like you're walking on eggshells—waiting for the next mood episode while simultaneously trying your best to keep things on an even keel for your mate. You may try to protect your partner from upsetting issues and situations, shouldering the load yourself to try to keep your loved one from being "triggered." Carrying an enormous burden like this can be extremely stressful, but you may be so tuned in to your mate's illness that you don't have time to think about its impact on you. Your emotional well-being, as a result, may fall by the wayside.

And that—your well-being—is the primary reason for my writing this book: to help people who don't have the illness meet (and, I hope, minimize) the challenges that come from having a loved one with bipolar disorder. Although many books have been written for people who have this disorder, almost none have been written expressly for you and others like you, the spouses and partners of those suffering with the illness.

In this book I've given you everything I know—from my patients' and their families' experiences, from the best research has to offer, and from the personal journey my husband and I have taken and continue to take—about living with and helping someone who has bipolar disorder. Not only will this book help you cope with your loved one's condition, it also will give you real strategies that you can use to help your mate get control over the mood swings. And by helping your mate, you will be helping yourself too.

My husband has seen me through numerous periods of depression and hypomania, yet he never seems ready to quit. I see the same response in the spouses of patients I work with. Out of all the couples I've met who are dealing with bipolar disorder, I can't think of a single one who has (at least to my knowledge) gotten a divorce. Obviously, my husband isn't the only one working through this illness with someone like me.

Since you too are living with and love someone who has bipolar disorder, I'm sure you're invested in doing everything you can to make the relationship work. At times I know this may seem impossible. If your partner has a severe form of the illness—getting into serious trouble during manic episodes or incapacitated or even worse when depressed—you may think you just can't take it anymore. But you know as well as I do that these periods don't last forever. And behind them is the person you love, the one you thought—and still hope—you'd be with forever.

You don't need to give up the dream of forever. As you will see in this book, there are a great many things you can do to help yourself and your partner to have that life. Although the path to achieving it may be rocky and have some obstacles, the jagged terrain will have footholds—real, solid places—where you can step, climb, and move forward together.

1

Does Someone You Love Have Bipolar Disorder?

Shelly is extremely worried about her fiancé, Peter, who has just been diagnosed with bipolar disorder. For the past couple of months he's been acting very strange, like a person she doesn't even know. His mood changes at the drop of a hat: one minute he's really cheerful and boisterous, the next irritable and angry and picking fights with her. He's hardly been sleeping, too, but instead of being exhausted he says he feels "wired" and that his thoughts are rushing through his head. Shelly believes this must be true because Peter is speaking really fast and tripping over his words; she can't even get a word in edgewise.

Shelly knows that Peter has had depressions in the past, but what he's going through now doesn't look like depression. What does it mean that Peter has "bipolar disorder"? Shelly thought they'd get married and have children one day, but now she's really concerned about their future.

Bipolar can be a very scary word, especially when it's used to describe someone you love. I know because as a psychologist I diagnose the illness in my practice and see the reactions of people and their families. I also know because my husband and I have had to hear the word applied to me.

When I was first told that I had bipolar disorder, I reacted with shock and disbelief. "I'm a manic–depressive?" I incredulously asked my doctor. "How is that possible? I have a husband, a career, and friends. There must be some mistake." But there was no mistake. My husband was equally stunned but, as is typical for him in the face of adversity, put on a brave face. Still, he couldn't hide the fact that, like Shelly, he was worried for our future.

Having diagnosed and treated bipolar disorder for so many years, it never ceases to amaze me how I "missed" my own diagnosis. I put the word *missed* in quotation marks because, in all honesty, I think I really did know what was going on with me; I just didn't want to face it. After all, nobody—including psychologists—wants to have bipolar disorder. But after years of blaming situations and other people for my mood swings, I finally had to face the undeniable truth—it was me, or rather my illness, that was to blame.

Externalizing blame is a way bipolar people try to make sense of what's happening to them. And it's also one of the reasons so many people with this illness go undiagnosed. They insist nothing is wrong with them and then refuse to see a mental health professional. Your partner even may say, "It's not me that has the problem; it's you!"

But you know it's not you. In fact, if you're like many spouses and partners of bipolar people, you have a temperament or personality type that's very different from the bipolar experience. If I had to put forth an educated guess (a guess based on 25 years of experience with bipolar people and their mates), I'd say that you're a fairly even-keeled, predictable person by nature, one who tends to "minimize" things as opposed to overreacting. Essentially you likely are, if you will, the pro-verbial calm in the middle of the storm. You also, if you are like a lot of the mates of bipolar individuals whom I've met, a "caregiver," a person who derives satisfaction from taking care of others. These qualities—your steadfastness and caregiving nature—may be partly why your mate picked you as a partner. It also may be partly why you picked your mate: you found your partner's personality exciting and the rela-tionship offered you an opportunity to express your nurturing side.

But I don't mean to overgeneralize. It's true that opposites don't always attract. You may, in fact, have been drawn to your partner's lively temperament because it resembles, in some ways, your own. In that case, if your partner is just moving into a depressed phase for the first time, you may feel like you've been blindsided, neither able nor willing to deal with the downside of mood swings.

Living with and loving somebody who has bipolar disorder is a daunting task. You may be the type of person who has the emotional strength to readily take on the difficulties that bipolar disorder presents. Or maybe you don't view yourself as particularly strong, steadfast, or as a natural nurturer; right now you just feel overwhelmed and confused. Either way, I expect that no one has given you guidance in how best to meet the challenges you've been handed.

Fortunately, because of both my professional and personal experience with this illness, I'm in a position to help. In this book I offer a wealth of practical strategies and suggestions for you to use at times when you want to help your mate but just don't know how, as well as emotional support for you during times when you just don't feel up to the task. But before getting to this, the very first step is to make sure your loved one really does have bipolar disorder and that the type of bipolar disorder has been identified correctly.

No one welcomes a diagnosis of bipolar disorder. It's a serious illness that has the potential to devastate individuals and wreak havoc in families. But if your loved one does have the illness, your opportunity to have the life you both want so badly rests on getting—and accepting (see Chapter 3)—the diagnosis.

Although it can feel like your life is over, being diagnosed with bipolar disorder really is a beginning. It's the beginning of making sense of the emotional roller coaster ride your loved one has been on, and it's the beginning of getting help—the right kind of help—for the illness. That's what happened for my husband and me, and it's what I expect will happen for you and your partner too.

Normal and Abnormal Moods

Manic–depressive illness—as bipolar disorder originally was called—was first described in the late 1800s by Emil Kraepelin, a German psychiatrist. If you've seen the movie *Mr. Jones* with Richard Gere, you have a good idea of Kraepelin's conceptualization of the disorder. The film shows a young man, untreated for his bipolar disorder, having ups and downs at the farthest ends of the continuum—suicidal depressions and psychotic (out of touch with reality) manias.

While the movie contains a good enactment of severe, psychotic manic–depressive illness, our understanding of the disorder today is much broader than this. The thinking now is that there is a *spectrum* of bipolar disorders that includes different forms of the illness, some of which are much milder and far less dramatic than the type Mr. Jones had. I am lucky (although at times in battling this illness I don't always feel so lucky) to have one of the milder, less disruptive forms of the disorder.

What Is a Mood?

Regardless of the form bipolar disorder takes (I'll get into the types later on), it always is first and foremost a disorder of *mood*. What is a mood? While there is no clear-cut or consensual definition of what a mood is, most professionals in this area probably would be comfortable with the idea that it's a pervasive, persistent emotional—or feeling— state. Feelings (happy, sad, angry, bored, jealous) can be fleeting, but when they last and color most everything we perceive and do, we're talking about a mood.

Certainly we all experience good and bad moods—periods when it feels like things are going well and others when we feel a little blue. Variations in mood may occur for no apparent reason, like waking up on the "right" or "wrong" side of the bed, or they can be reactions to events, like when something positive or negative happens.

For people with bipolar disorder, changes in mood go way beyond this norm. Instead of giving them a pleasant feeling of well-being, the ups can make them feel too "high" or irritable, causing difficulty in their relationships or getting them into trouble. During the down periods they are way down—severely depressed, sometimes even to the point of near incapacitation or preoccupation with suicide. When moods are extreme and go in two different directions like this— "up," the manic or hypomanic (mildly manic) state, and "down," the depressed state—bipolar disorder likely is to blame.

What Do Changes in Mood Look Like during Mania and Hypomania?

The mood that is experienced during mania and hypomania is *elevated* or *irritable*, or, as for Peter, who I talked about at the beginning of this chapter, both. At its extreme, an elevated mood can be euphoric, a state of elation or ecstasy. This feeling has been described by some of my patients as similar to what it feels like to fall in love. Sometimes the mood is "higher" than normal—it's elevated, "too happy"—but not to the point of euphoria. For me it's what I'd describe as very "upbeat."

During manic or hypomanic times your partner may be very jovial, joking around in a way that's not typical for him (like being silly or making puns), smiling and laughing a lot (more than usual), singing out loud (possibly even when no music is playing), or walking with an unusual gait, like with a skip or at a very quick pace. You might hear comments from your partner about how "wonderful" things are or how "really great" he feels even though nothing in particular has happened.

An elevated mood can, however, change to an irritable, angry mood, or even rage in some bipolar individuals, or the mood disturbance can be entirely irritable with no "high." You may find your partner gets into altercations easily, not just with you but possibly with strangers as well, and may even seem to be looking for fights. Your partner may be insulting to others (or, on the other hand, feel easily insulted or slighted) or yell or scream readily. Sometimes the belligerence turns from verbal to physical, and your mate can end up in physical confrontations that may result in run-ins with the law. For others with the disorder anger is not this intense, but they consistently are very easily irritated or annoyed and extremely edgy. When I get this way, my husband says that I'm "impossible to talk to."

What Does a Depressed Mood Look Like?

By contrast, the predominant mood in depression is sadness. People have different ways of communicating this feeling. Your mate may use the word "sad" or say she is feeling "depressed," "low," "blue," or "down in the dumps." Sometimes, instead, the feeling is described as emptiness, numbness, or extreme boredom. Some people say the experience is like being trapped in a tunnel with no light at the end. Or a person may say it feels like there's a black cloud or veil over his head. Your mate may describe feeling emotional pain that's unendurable, which patients have described to me as feeling similar to having one's heart "broken." Instead of verbalizing these feelings, your partner may exhibit tearfulness as a sign of what's going on inside.

Abnormal moods, while necessary, do not by themselves indicate that someone has bipolar disorder. To have bipolar disorder, a person must have *mood episodes*—distinct periods of time that are marked not just by abnormal mood but by other symptoms as well.

Manic and Hypomanic Episodes

The symptoms, including abnormal mood, of mania and hypomania are listed in the sidebar on the facing page.

According to our psychiatric diagnostic system (from the American Psychiatric Association's *Diagnostic and Statistical Manual of Mental Disorders*, which had its last major revision—*DSM-IV*—in 1994), manic and hypomanic episodes are defined by a persistently elevated or irritable mood plus three or four of the other symptoms listed in the sidebar: three symptoms if the mood is elevated, four symptoms if the mood is irritable. Also, all of the symptoms must occur during the same time period. For a hypomanic episode, the symptoms must have persisted for at least 4 days; for a manic episode, 7 days unless there has been a hospitalization, in which case any length of time counts as an episode.

Mania and Hypomania: What's the Difference?

As you can see from the sidebar, the symptoms of manic and hypomanic episodes are exactly the same. You might be wondering, then, what the difference is. Actually, there are three differences you should know about. First, hypomanic episodes do not interfere with functioning—like the ability to work or to relate to other people—to the extent that manic episodes do. For instance, in my case, as I'll talk about in more detail later on, my hypomania does not negatively impact my work life.

Second, hypomanic episodes never, by definition, contain psychotic features—that is, delusions (irrational, unfounded fixed beliefs) or hallucinations (hearing, seeing, smelling, or feeling something that is not there)—while manic episodes frequently do. Third, and finally, hypomanic episodes never necessitate a hospitalization; manic episodes, on the other hand, sometimes do, to prevent the person from harming him- or herself or someone else (see Chapter 8).

Actually, hypomanic episodes can be extremely pleasant for peo-

Symptoms of Mania and Hypomania

- An elevated or irritable mood (or both)
- Extreme self-confidence or an exaggerated sense of self-importance
- Reduced need for sleep
- Talkativeness or "pressured" speech (like the person can't get the words out fast enough)
- Racing thoughts
- Distractibility
- Increased productivity at home, school, or work; increased sociability and/or sexuality; physical agitation (restless, pacing, jumping out of his or her skin)
- Risky behaviors that display impulsivity and/or poor judgment, like spending sprees, excessive gambling, driving while intoxicated, extramarital affairs, or getting involved in "get rich quick" schemes

ple whose moods are more elevated than irritable and who are not plagued by the consequences of serious risk-taking behavior. And it's not only pleasant for the individual who is experiencing such a mood. Hypomanic moods can be infectious. Other people often love being around gregarious, witty, self-confident individuals whose "feel goods" seem to rub off on them. (I believe, in fact, that it was my hypomanic self that my husband fell in love with and that this is the self he still sees when he pictures me in his mind.)

To better understand what mania and hypomania are like, let's look at some of the things spouses and partners of people who are having these kinds of episodes have had to say about their mates:

"My wife is constantly tooting her own horn, telling me and other people how great she really is. This is so unlike her!"

Increased self-confidence or an exaggerated sense of self-importance ("grandiosity") is common in manic and hypomanic states. In mania the grandiosity may become of delusional proportion, where the person believes he or she has some special power or knowledge, or is—or has a significant relationship to—a very important or famous person.

"He's sleeping only 4 hours a night but is filled with energy."

A decreased need for sleep—not just *getting* less sleep but *needing* less sleep—is very characteristic of mania and hypomania. In mania the sleep disturbance usually is more profound (very little or no sleep) than in hypomania.

"My wife seems to get distracted by the littlest thing."

Getting easily distracted by extraneous stimuli in the environment can occur during manic and hypomanic episodes. Your mate may have trouble with concentration because he or she loses focus easily, attending to unimportant sights and sounds.

"He's usually a very careful driver, but now he's speeding all the time and driving very offensively and aggressively."

Manic and hypomanic people are, let me say, in an "accelerated mode." They may think faster, talk faster, walk faster, and, as in this case, drive faster. In fact, you may hear your partner say that things aren't happening fast enough, encouraging you to "move along" more quickly in whatever you are doing.

The reckless road behavior is, though, not just a reflection of the faster pace that's present in mania and hypomania. It's a risky behavior that has the potential for negative consequences—traffic tickets, automobile accidents, or even worse.

"My wife has become obsessed with work, but I have to say she's getting a lot done."

Increased productivity—at home, school, or work—can be a benefit of hypomania, as long as it remains goal directed (focused on a specific worthwhile purpose) and doesn't become *too* obsessive (where other responsibilities are ignored because of overinvolvement in a single activity).

"He's spending money like it's water."

Spending too much money—that is, spending that's above one's means—is a common concern of the mates of bipolar people. During manic and hypomanic episodes your partner may go on spending sprees or engage in excessive gambling. Like reckless driving and other types of risky activities, this is an impulsive behavior that reflects bad judgment, the consequences of which can be painful and long lasting (the accumulation of large debts).

"She's calling lots of people she hasn't talked to in years."

Increased sociability and gregariousness frequently occur in manic and hypomanic states. You may notice that your partner is e-mailing an abundance of people or talking excessively on the phone, or making many more social plans than usual. Sometimes the increased gregariousness takes an inappropriate turn—being overfriendly to strangers or making phone calls in the middle of the night.

"His sex drive has gone way up."

Some people have an increased libido when manic or hypomanic. During these times your mate may want more frequent sexual contact with you. It's also not uncommon for men, in particular, to compulsively visit strip clubs or become excessively involved with pornography. Having extramarital affairs is a sexually motivated risk-taking behavior that also can occur (I'll talk more about this in Chapter 8).

"She's very restless, pacing, can't sit still, wringing her hands."

Physical agitation can occur in both manic and hypomanic states, but it's likely to be more severe in mania. For example, during hypomania your mate may be very fidgety and complain of feeling restless but can sit in one spot for a period of time. Manic agitation is harder to miss—your partner may be pacing the floors nonstop, unable to sit in one place for very long, and/or wringing her hands.

"My husband has all of a sudden become a neat freak, cleaning the house even in the middle of the night."

As I said earlier, increased productivity—in the home, at school, or at work—is a sign that a manic or hypomanic episode may be under way. Remember, manic and hypomanic people are on a fast clock—if they aren't easily distracted and their thinking isn't really impaired, they can get a lot done in surprisingly little time. In this man's case, though, he's having trouble sleeping and is wound up and full of energy at the wrong time of the day—that's why he's doing housework in the wee hours of the morning.

"She says that her thoughts are coming too fast."

People who are manic or hypomanic often complain of racing thoughts, ideas, or images (pictures in their heads). Your partner may describe this as like an audiotape/CD or videotape/DVD being played on fast forward. The racing thoughts may show up as accelerated speech too (see page 17).

"He's talking way faster than is normal for him, like he's taking speed."

The presence of pressured speech—the need to talk a lot and to do so quickly—is a telltale sign of mania and hypomania and may go hand in hand with racing thoughts (fast thoughts, fast talk). As for Peter, introduced at the beginning of this chapter, it's not unusual for people to end up tripping over their own words. In severe cases the speech can be so rapid that it's hard to follow what the person is saying. In either event it's almost impossible to have a two-way conversation with someone who is like this; the nonstop talking doesn't allow for dialogue.

Although I really don't have full-blown hypomanic episodes anymore because of the medication that I take (more on medication in Chapter 4), I can remember what they were like. As I said earlier, my mood generally was upbeat, although I would become irritable if I was challenged or something didn't go my way. For instance, I remember getting really angry (*livid* probably would be a better word) and raising my voice at a clerk in a bookstore because a book of mine that had just been published was in boxes rather than on the shelves.

Also during these periods I was very self-confident, energetic (exercising), sociable (calling old friends), and creative (I had lots of ideas for decorating my home, new research studies, new books, etc.). I was a version of myself that I really liked and, as I said before, one my husband liked too. (Do my husband and I miss the highs that my medication has dampened? In some ways we both do. But since "what goes up must come down," we agree that the highs definitely weren't worth the lows that inevitably followed.)

During hypomanic episodes I also found that my thinking had more clarity and that I was more productive. In other words, my hypomania actually was beneficial to my work. And I'm not alone in this— I've had many bipolar colleagues and patients tell me they've experienced the same thing.

But certainly not all hypomanias are like this. For some people persistently irritable, angry moods negatively affect relationships, both at home and at work. Trouble with thinking, because of racing thoughts and/or distractibility, impairs the ability to meet responsibilities (attending to children, performing at one's job, taking care of the home). Impulsivity and poor judgment lead people to do things that can come back to haunt them.

Manias are even more impairing. By definition, the mood disturbance and accompanying symptoms are severe enough to cause *marked* impairment in functioning (at work or as a homemaker or in a person's usual social activities or relationships). And remember, people who are manic can have psychotic symptoms—delusions or hallucinations—too. Manic delusions and hallucinations often revolve around themes of inflated self-worth (having special or supernatural powers, taking on the identity of someone seen as having more status, believing there is a special relationship to a deity or famous person), or else are persecutory, what most people would call "paranoid."

Now that you have a good idea of what mania and hypomania are like, let's talk about the other side of the coin, depressive episodes.

Depressive Episodes

The symptoms of depression, including abnormal mood, are listed in the sidebar below.

Symptoms of Depression

- Depressed mood
- Loss of interest in or pleasure from all, or almost all, activities
- Appetite disturbance or weight loss or weight gain
- Trouble sleeping or sleeping too much
- Physical agitation or a slowdown
- Feelings of worthlessness or guilt (excessive or inappropriate self-blame)
- Feeling tired most of the time or without energy
- Slowed thinking, difficulty concentrating, or inability to make decisions
- Repeated thoughts about death or suicide or a suicide attempt

---

A depressive episode is defined by the presence of five of the symptoms—one of which has to be depressed mood or loss of interest in activities—all at once, nearly every day for at least 2 weeks. Also, the symptoms must either cause a great deal of distress to the person or interfere with some important area of functioning, like performance at work or school or relationships with others (like with you).

Now that you know what constitutes a depressive episode, let's look at some things partners and spouses of people experiencing it have had to say:

"My husband doesn't want to do anything anymore. He's completely lost interest in the things he used to like to do."

A loss of interest in (and pleasure from) one's usual activities is a very common feature of depression. Your mate may complain that the things he liked to do are now "boring," that they just don't seem interesting or important anymore. Or the loss of interest in things can be part of a general state of inertia that depressed people frequently experience (for example, it may take inordinate effort to do anything, even something as simple as taking a shower). The loss of interest and inertia can extend to social interactions too, resulting in your mate's withdrawing from you and other people. Your partner may experience a lowered libido and, possibly, sexual dysfunction (erectile dysfunction in men; inability to have an orgasm in women).

"My wife is hardly eating, and she's lost a ton of weight."

Decreased appetite and (unintended) weight loss are common symptoms of depression, although increased appetite and weight gain can occur instead. Those who have an increased appetite may crave specific types of foods, like carbohydrates or sweets.

"He's waking up early in the morning, hours before he has to get up."

A sleep disturbance is a frequent symptom of depression. There can be either decreased sleep—trouble falling asleep, trouble staying asleep, or waking up earlier than usual—or increased sleep, referred to as *hypersomnia*. In addition to sleeping too long at night, people with hypersomnia may take naps during the day. Even when not sleeping, often a depressed person develops a "love affair" with his bed, spending inordinate amounts of time there.

*"My wife has always been a decisive person. Now she can't
even make the smallest of decisions."*

People who are depressed often have trouble with their thinking. They
may think more slowly (and, possibly, as a result, have slowed speech),
have trouble concentrating or, like this man's wife did, become very
indecisive. Your mate also may complain of being easily distracted or
of having memory problems.

*"My fiancé is constantly complaining of being tired and, to
tell you the truth, he acts like he is, like he has no energy at all."*

Feeling fatigued all the time, even though one is getting enough sleep,
is a common feature of depression. People also can appear physically
slowed—for instance, talking or walking more slowly than is usual for
them. (The opposite—being physically agitated—can occur instead; if
your mate is pacing or having trouble sitting still, it's a good bet that
this is what's happening.)

"She's constantly putting herself down."

Feelings of worthlessness and self-hatred frequently are part of depression. Your partner also, or instead, may feel guilty and to blame for
things that are not her fault or may dwell excessively on being to blame
for a certain situation, for instance, being a burden to you because of
the depression.

*"My husband says over and over again that he wishes he
were dead."*

Wishes to be dead and, even more tragically, acts of self-harm are not
unusual when people are depressed (see Chapter 2). These thoughts
and acts usually are fueled by feelings of hopelessness—people believing that the emotional pain they have will never come to an end. (I'll
talk about what to do in a situation like this in Chapters 8 and 9.)

I've had many depressed episodes during the course of my bipolar
illness. But at this point in my life, because I'm kind of used to them,
have tools to deal with them, and know they'll end, and because they
are modulated to a significant extent by my family environment and
the medications I take, I approach the days that I'm in a down cycle,
at least initially when I start each day, with hope.

This is not, however, the way I felt when I was much younger, or the way most depressed people feel. Hopefulness is not characteristic of depression and probably is not, at least at the present time (though my expectation is that things will get much better as you and your partner use the strategies and other advice in this book), the way your partner would describe his depressions. Quite to the contrary, as I said before, *hopelessness* is something many depressed people feel, and I remember feeling it intensely during my teens and my 20s. During those times, although I never attempted suicide, I recall despair so strong that all I wished for was to close my eyes, go to sleep, and not wake up again. (As I'm writing this it's hard for me to believe that this once was true, because, thankfully, I haven't felt that way for a very long time.)

When a person is depressed, perceptions get distorted and the past, the present, and the future all look bleak—nothing good has ever happened or will ever happen. Things actually look different too. The world looks gray—colors seem to fade (this is the opposite of the manic or hypomanic state, where, for many, colors seem much brighter).

As opposed to mania and hypomania, in depression everything can feel slowed down. Thinking may be slowed, speech is slowed, and movement is slowed. Your partner may describe feeling very heavy or like a weight is pressing down on her. Time seems to go more slowly, too—each hour is like an eternity.

Depressive episodes, like manic episodes, can have psychotic features. Often the delusions and hallucinations are related to depressive themes, like guilt, personal shortcomings, or deserving punishment (for example, "I'm so bad that God is punishing me").

Mixed Episodes

Mania, hypomania, and depression are three kinds of mood episodes your loved one is likely to experience, but you should know that many people—about 40% of individuals who have bipolar disorder—have mixed episodes, which consist of both manic and depressed symptoms. That is, during mixed episodes the criteria for mania and depression are met *during the same time period.*

Gwen, a 39-year-old homemaker with bipolar disorder, is in a mixed episode. Her husband says her mood changes rapidly from cheerful and laughing to sad and crying and then back to cheerful and laughing again. She has symptoms of mania—a need for less sleep, racing thoughts, "pressured" speech—and she's physically agitated, but she also has symptoms of depression: less appetite, loss of interest in her usual activities, and suicidal thoughts.

In fact, Gwen exemplifies three things that are common to mixed episodes: rapidly alternating moods, physical agitation, and suicidal thoughts.

Mixed episodes can be tricky to pinpoint. Because of the presence of depressed symptoms, your partner could be diagnosed incorrectly as having depression. You definitely don't want this to happen, because the treatment of depression is different from the treatment of mixed episodes that are part of bipolar disorder. In fact, research has shown that antidepressant medications commonly used to treat depression may precipitate the development of mixed episodes in people who have bipolar tendencies. They've also been shown to trigger "rapid cycling" in bipolar disorder, that is, to shorten the time between mood episodes so that four or more (manic, hypomanic, mixed, or depressed episodes) occur in a year's time.

The Diagnosis: Type I and Type II Bipolar Disorder

Mood episodes form the basis for diagnosing bipolar disorder, and the types of episodes your partner experiences determine which one of two possible diagnoses applies to your mate. Bipolar type I ("bipolar I") indicates that there has been at least one manic or mixed episode. Bipolar type II ("bipolar II") is the type of bipolar disorder that I have. It means that I have a history of hypomanic episodes and episodes of depression but no manic or mixed episodes.

It's important to understand that if your spouse has had depressive episodes but no manic or hypomanic (or mixed) episodes, by definition she doesn't have bipolar disorder. Instead, the appropriate diagnosis would be *major depressive disorder*. Although bipolar depression and "unipolar depression" (a term used to describe depressions where there is no history of mania, mixed, or hypomania) share similar qualities, the distinction between the two is important particularly because of the implications for treatment. As I said before, this is especially true with regard to medication. The pharmacological treatment of major depression is different from the approach taken for manic–depression, even though manic–depression includes, at times, depressive episodes.

Because manic and mixed episodes are, by definition, more severe than hypomanic episodes, people who have bipolar I disorder may be more incapacitated by their illness than people who have bipolar II disorder. I say "may be more incapacitated" because individuals with both types of the disorder can suffer equally severe episodes of depression. Remember, the distinction between the two conditions is based on the presence (or absence) of manic and mixed episodes only.

Even people who have the same type of bipolar illness may differ in terms of their symptoms and the effects the illness has on their lives. That's why for both bipolar I and bipolar II the severity of the condition is designated as "mild," "moderate," or "severe." Todd has a mild version of bipolar I disorder—he's never had psychotic symptoms, been suicidal, or been hospitalized for the disorder. And as difficult as it sometimes is, he can still work. Elizabeth, on the other hand, has a severe form of bipolar I disorder. She experiences horrible hallucinations during episodes and has tried to hurt her husband on several occasions. She's been hospitalized a number of times and can no longer work.

Ben and Kayla both have bipolar II disorder, but that's where the similarity ends. Ben has had countless severe and lengthy depressions, while Kayla has had only one mild episode of depression, which lasted for just a couple of months. Ben also, unlike Kayla, gets into trouble when he's hypomanic because of his risk taking—uncontrolled gambling, extramarital affairs, and use of street drugs like cocaine. (Bipolar disorder frequently coexists with substance abuse, a topic we'll talk about later in this chapter and again, at length, in Chapters 7 and 8.) Kayla, on the other hand, becomes very focused and productive during her hypomanic periods.

Cyclothymic Disorder

Although cyclothymic disorder is not exactly considered a type of bipolar disorder, the symptom picture, which includes ups and downs, makes it something you should know about. *Cyclothymic disorder* involves periods of hypomanic symptoms that alternate with periods of depressive symptoms, but the depressive symptoms do not meet the full criteria for a depressive episode. An example of this would be if your mate had only three, rather than the required five, symptoms of depression, or if the depressive symptoms weren't present nearly every day. One more thing about cyclothymic disorder is that, unlike bipolar disorder, the condition must be present for *at least 2 years* before it can be diagnosed.

If your partner has cyclothymia and not bipolar disorder, it's still very important for you to read this book. Much of the information contained in these chapters can be applied to you and your partner just as well as it can be applied to bipolar disorder. Also, since research shows that about one-third of people with cyclothymic disorder go on to develop bipolar II disorder (that's not to say that your loved one will be one of those who goes on to develop bipolar disorder; it just means that the odds are greater than for someone who never has had cyclothymia), using the tools provided in later chapters also may help to prevent your partner's mild mood swing problem from worsening and developing into a more severe mood swing problem.

I also want to briefly talk about "seasonal affective disorder." You may have heard the term used in the media—in magazine or newspaper articles or on television. The term is used to describe depressive symptoms people experience during certain seasons, most commonly during winter months ("winter blues") in northern states.

I had the winter blues when I lived in a northern climate. And since I knew that the treatment for it was light therapy, I used to go to a tanning booth to get ultraviolet light (and also get a nice golden tan) to pick up my mood. Ultimately, part of my decision to move to Florida was based on my thinking that my depressions would go away if I were in a sunnier climate. Unfortunately, since what I actually had was bipolar disorder, moving to Florida wasn't the answer.

But I bring up seasonal affective disorder because there are studies that suggest the condition predisposes people to develop cyclothymia and/or bipolar disorder. Because of this, if your partner is experiencing this problem, please go ahead and use the methods described later in this book for alleviating depression. Improving the mood problem that exists today not only may help now but also may help prevent future, more severe mood problems down the road.

Bipolar Disorder or Major Depression?

Although the symptoms of mania and depression listed in the side-bars on pages 13 and 17 may seem clear and straightforward, making the diagnosis of bipolar disorder is not always easy. People who have hypomanic episodes, nonpsychotic, manic episodes with an irritable (as opposed to an elevated) mood, or mixed episodes, sometimes end up being diagnosed as having major depression when that's really only half of the story.

I know this happens not only because of the countless number of patients with mood disorders I've worked with over the years, but also because of how this issue played out in my own life. Although examining my history makes it clear that I've suffered from bipolar disorder since adolescence, all of the doctors I saw through my teens, 20s, and early 30s diagnosed me as having depression—the hypo-manic episodes (which meant my diagnosis should have been bipolar II disorder) were missed. I actually didn't get the correct diagnosis (and, consequently, didn't get the right kind of help for my condition) until my mid-30s.

One likely reason that my hypomanic episodes were missed is that I sought treatment only at times when I was depressed, not when I was hypomanic. And apparently I'm not alone in this. Research shows that people with bipolar disorder tend to seek out professional help when depressed but, on the other hand, are *unlikely* to go see a doctor when manic or hypomanic (unless someone else brings them in). As a result, doctors usually see patients when they're in depressions, and unless they probe carefully for past periods of mania or hypomania they can end up giving the diagnosis of major depression, as in my case, instead of bipolar disorder. (This also may be part of the reason why *it takes an average of 8 years from the onset of bipolar disorder to the diagnosis.*)

Even when doctors probe for past episodes of mania or hypoma-nia, they can come up "empty-handed" because bipolar patients often aren't good historians when it comes to chronicling their "up" periods. (This is one of the reasons your input can be so valuable to the diagnostic process, a subject I discuss at length in Chapter 5.)

Your mate may not tell the doctor about manic or hypomanic symptoms because she is embarrassed to share this information, even with a mental health professional. Mismanaging money, adultery, substance abuse, and getting in trouble with the law aren't behaviors that people are proud of and want to talk about. You might be surprised to know how often psychiatrists and psychologists are unaware that things like this are occurring in their patients' lives—that is, until they have input from a close family member; then the pieces of the puzzle fall into place.

This is what happened to 30-year-old Dana, who never told her psychiatrist about her three DUIs (driving under the influence) and over-the-top spending sprees. It wasn't until her husband, Mark, accompanied her to an appointment and shared this information that the doctor began to get a picture of what was really going on, that Dana had another side—a manic side—to her mood problem.

Sometimes it's not that people are concealing information from their doctors; it's that they genuinely are unaware of or misinterpret the manic or hypomanic side of their mood swings. For example, if your loved one generally has a happy, elevated mood during hypomanic or nonpsychotic, manic episodes, he (and you too) may mistake the up times as his "true" or normal self (the depressed times, on the other hand, being the "not true" or ill self), and, as a result, not report it to the doctor. It's not hard to see how this happens—it makes sense that people tend to identify more with their upbeat, gregarious, creative, energetic sides than their depressed sides. People who have very few or no periods of normal mood—that is, who alternate largely between periods of high and low moods—are especially likely to interpret their highs in this way.

A different reason people with bipolar disorder can be diagnosed as having major depression can lie in the general approach some doctors take to diagnosing their patients—diagnosing the disorder that's "of least consequence," that is, the one that's least difficult for the patient to hear about and accept. In the case of bipolar disorder, a psychiatrist or a psychologist may suspect or know that a patient has the illness but instead label the problem as major depression, because it's less stigmatizing and has a better prognosis associated with it.

In fact, this is what happened to a new patient of mine, 39-year-old Kafi. Prior to meeting Kafi I consulted with his psychiatrist, who confirmed that he was in a manic episode of bipolar disorder. But when I met with Kafi and his wife to discuss things they might do to help keep Kafi's bipolar disorder under control, the couple told me that the problem wasn't bipolar disorder. The psychiatrist had told them the diagnosis was major depression.

Although situations like this are very much in the minority, they do happen, and I wanted to share this with you. (And please know that I'm not trying to say anything negative about psychiatrists. Psychologists, and other mental health professionals, can do this too.) Although it's true that nobody wants to have bipolar disorder, individuals should know their diagnoses so that they can learn about their illness and ways they can help themselves. Also, knowing about the course, prognosis, and heritability of the disorder can assist people and their mates in making good decisions for their futures.

Could My Partner Have Something Else?

Several psychiatric disorders have symptoms that overlap with the symptoms of bipolar disorder and, consequently, can lead to diagnostic uncertainty. I'll try to clarify the differences between them and bipolar disorder in the following discussion.

Schizophrenia

Schizophrenia is one psychiatric condition that's frequently confused with bipolar I disorder. The acute phase of schizophrenia—when people often have hallucinations and/or delusions—can look similar to a manic episode with psychotic features. The difference between them, however, is twofold.

First, schizophrenia has a different type of history and course than manic–depressive illness: schizophrenia is chronic and unremitting (the person is never really well), while bipolar disorder is episodic. Second, in schizophrenia the hallucinations and delusions tend to be rather bizarre—like people thinking other people can read their minds. In contrast, hallucinations and delusions that occur in a psychotic mania or depression tend to be less bizarre and more mood-congruent. By mood-congruent I mean that whatever the psychosis is about goes along with the individual's mood, like grandiose delusions or hallucinations when manic. For example, when she's manic Deanna has a recurrent delusion that she's God—Jesus Christ—himself. During his recent manic episode, Taylor felt light as the air—so light that he thought he could fly.

However, it's not unusual for people with psychotic manias to have paranoid delusions or hallucinations. This can be very difficult to distinguish from paranoid schizophrenia. Here the history of the mood problems relative to the history of the psychosis can help to clarify the diagnostic picture—in mania, the psychosis occurs only during the mood episode, whereas in paranoid schizophrenia the mood disturbance is relatively brief in comparison to the length of time the delusions or hallucinations have persisted.

I can't tell you how many times the spouses of bipolar patients have asked me whether their partners really have schizophrenia. They ask me this out of fear—while it's true nobody wants to have bipolar disorder, people want to have schizophrenia even less. In situations like this it's absolutely best to leave this determination to your doctor. If you don't have ample confidence in your doctor, please find another one, or at least get a second opinion. (See Chapter 4 for how to find the right doctor.)

Schizoaffective Disorder

Schizoaffective disorder, which includes both schizophrenic symptoms and a mood episode, can be even more difficult to distinguish from bipolar I disorder than schizophrenia is. The main difference between the two is that for schizoaffective disorder there must be, at some point during the illness, a period of at least 2 weeks when hallucinations or delusions are present *in the absence of* prominent mood symptoms. This, of course, contrasts with bipolar episodes that have psychotic features, where the hallucinations or delusions occur only during a manic, mixed, or depressed state.

If your significant other has bipolar disorder, you certainly don't want him misdiagnosed as having schizophrenia or schizoaffective disorder, and, conversely, if your loved one really has one of these two disorders, you don't want him misdiagnosed as having bipolar disorder. The treatments and the prognoses for these illnesses differ. So if you have a concern like this, I strongly urge you to seek a second opinion from another doctor, one who has a reputation as having expertise in this area.

Personality Disorder

Personality disorders are persistent, maladaptive emotional responses and behavior that stem from a distorted view of oneself and the world (other people and events). They begin in adolescence or early adulthood and cause the individuals who have them distress and/or impair their functioning.

Certain types of personality disorders (there are 10 different types) can be difficult to distinguish from bipolar disorder. To further complicate matters, personality disorders frequently coexist with bipolar disorder.

Although it is beyond the scope of this book to discuss all, or even several, of the personality disorders in detail, there is one personality disorder that I want to mention by name: borderline personality disorder. A number of its features are quite similar to experiences bipolar people have: mood instability, impulsivity (engaging in risky behavior that has the potential for painful consequences), suicidal thoughts and behavior, paranoid thoughts, and intense anger.

A key difference between bipolar disorder and borderline personality disorder (although, as I said before, they can coexist) is that bipolar disorder is an episodic illness while borderline personality disorder is, like all personality disorders, stable and ever present across time (for example, the person always suffers from unstable moods and is always impulsive). However, with that being said, I need to say that mixed episodes and the rapid-cycling form of bipolar illness—where there is, if you will, a stable form of instability—can look increasingly like borderline personality disorder.

Since even experienced clinicians can have trouble differentiating between the two conditions, I again urge you to see someone who specializes in diagnosing bipolar disorder so you're sure what you're up against (see Chapter 4 for how to go about finding the right doctor).

Personality Traits

I find that sometimes the partners and spouses of people with bipolar disorder will acknowledge that their mates have "personality issues," but they can't see that the situation is more serious than this, that it is a mental health problem. It's possible that you, too, view your loved one's behavior in this way. You may think of your mate as just being "difficult"—particularly if she has a relatively mild version of bipolar disorder—rather than as someone who has an illness.

You may say, "My wife is just a yeller," but if you find that during certain times—times when your spouse is easily irritated and angry— some of the other symptoms listed in the sidebar for manic and hypo- manic episodes (see page 13) are present, then you might want to con- sider the possibility of bipolar disorder, particularly if there is a history of depression too.

Richard loves his wife of 15 years but admits she has some person- ality traits that are very hard to live with. Carolyn is very moody and flies off the handle at the littlest thing. At times she's very aggressive— demanding, critical, and argumentative—while at other times she's oversensitive and easily hurt. There also are instances when she's so consumed with emotion that she's irrational and unpredictable. Other times she's completely the opposite: withdrawn and depressed.

If Richard and Carolyn had gone to see a mental health profes- sional, they might have discovered that Carolyn has a mild form of rapid-cycling bipolar II disorder and that there are treatment options that could have made both their lives much better. But since they haven't, they continue to live with Carolyn's "difficult" personality and they probably will for the rest of their marriage.

Please don't let this happen to you and your loved one. Mood swings—to the extent that Carolyn has them—are not normal. If something like this is going on in your home, it's in the interest of your entire family for you to try to persuade your mate to at least be evalu- ated by a mental health professional. Give yourself and your partner the opportunity for a better future.

Substance Abuse

People with bipolar disorder, especially those who aren't being treated for their conditions, frequently abuse substances—alcohol, prescrip- tion drugs, and/or street drugs. I discuss this problem at length in Chapters 7 and 8, but in terms of the diagnostic issues it raises, let me say that it really isn't possible to diagnose any type of mood disor- der with certainty when a person is habitually "under the influence." That's because substance abuse creates mood swings and unpredict- able behavior. For this reason, your partner is going to need to be "clean and sober" before the diagnosis of bipolar disorder can be made with certainty. Again, I point you to Chapters 7 and 8 to see how to handle substance abuse.

By now you should have a pretty good idea whether your loved one has bipolar disorder. But what does this mean for your partner and you in the near and long term? The next chapter will give you some idea of what the future may bring.

What You Can Expect

The Course of Bipolar Illness

Carlos is extremely worried. His wife, Yvonne, is about to give birth to their first child. While for most people this would be an exciting time, it's a time of great concern for this couple because of Yvonne's bipolar disorder.

Yvonne's doctors agreed that she should discontinue her medications during her pregnancy. But while doing so has kept her unborn child from possible harm, it has left Yvonne herself "unprotected." The danger to Yvonne is increased because, like all bipolar women, she is at greatest risk for a mood episode right after giving birth.

Will Yvonne be okay and able to care for their newborn? What will her husband do if her mood problem recurs and she can't function? Carlos anxiously waits to see what the future will bring.

One of the most difficult aspects of living with bipolar disorder, for both the person who has the disorder and that person's significant other, is the uncertainty surrounding the recurrence of mood episodes. Will your partner have another manic or depressive episode? If so, when?

As you'll see in this chapter, the course of bipolar disorder is extremely variable. Some people have mood episodes like clockwork—

31

for example, according to the seasons or following certain types of stressful or physically challenging life events (like having a baby), while for others episodes seem to appear "out of the blue"; there may be a trigger, but it can't be identified. Some bipolar individuals find they're battling mood episodes most of the time, having very few or no periods of normal mood, while others go for years or even decades without any problems.

The unpredictable nature of this illness can be a huge obstacle to making plans. If your partner doesn't know how she will be next week, next month, or next year, she may find it hard to make commitments. And since most everything we do is based on future plans, from our social lives ("Let's have dinner next Saturday") to work projects ("The report is due next month") and even vacation times ("We'll go to Vermont in the summer"), the potential impact of bipolar disorder on families' lives can be enormous.

Uncertainty about the future may cause you to feel like you're in limbo, unable to move forward for fear that the illness will spring up and stop you and your mate right in your tracks. Or despite your efforts to be understanding, you may be frustrated with your partner's continuing to say "no" to doing things you used to do together before she was ill or when she was feeling better. If your loved one has been very ill for quite some time, maybe you've been disappointed on so many occasions that you no longer have hope for things to improve.

The good news, though—and there is good news—is that there are very effective treatments and self-help strategies, some of which didn't exist even a decade ago, that can boost confidence and security about the future for both you and your partner. By stabilizing mood, your mate will be better able to make plans without the anxious anticipation and hesitation that comes from not knowing how he will be when it comes time to fulfill them.

In this chapter I'll be talking about factors that influence the course of bipolar disorder. Some of these—like age at onset of the illness and gender—are set and can't be changed, but others, like exposure to certain triggers and willingness to take medication as a preventive, are within your mate's reach. By paying close attention to what *can* be changed, you and your partner will be in a position to help control this illness, positively affecting your loved one's course and your future together.

How Often Will My Partner Have Mood Episodes?

Bipolar disorder is a recurrent disorder with multiple episodes being the rule rather than the exception. In fact we know that *almost all individuals who have this illness—more than 90%—will go on to have future mood episodes.* So the odds of your loved one's having a recurrence of the illness are high.

Although we know it's extremely likely that your mate will have more mood episodes, no one can tell you the exact number your partner will have over time or how often they'll occur. What we do know is that *without medication people have on the average of four episodes in 10 years, with 80% of individuals having a recurrence within 3 years and many much sooner.*

I know these are difficult pieces of information to digest. They are particularly hard to hear if your mate is newly ill or newly diagnosed and you were hoping that "the worst" was over, that your loved one might be better from here on out. While I can't tell you that because, unfortunately, it may not be true, I can tell you that there are many factors that affect the frequency of mood episodes, many of which you and your mate have the potential to control.

Factors That Decrease the Frequency of Episodes

As you'll see in the second half of this book, each of the following plays a role in decreasing the chances that your partner will have another mood episode:

- Getting professional help—medication and psychological treatment
- Being alert for potential triggers of mood episodes
- Adhering to a daily routine, including keeping a regular sleep–wake cycle
- Being vigilant for early warning signs of a mood disturbance so that the problem can be nipped in the bud before it blossoms into a full-blown mood episode

There's a reason that I listed getting professional help first in the preceding list: *the single largest contributor to remaining free of mood disturbance is taking medication as a prophylaxis* (that is, a preventive). I discuss this further in Chapters 4 and 6.

Breakthrough Episodes

You need to know that even on medication (and with adherence to the other methods for staying well) your partner can have "breakthrough" episodes of illness. This can happen even when someone has been successfully stabilized for a long time. That's why you and your mate need to watch out for being lulled into a false sense of security, thinking the disorder has gone away or "been cured" (thinking that, as I'll discuss in Chapter 6, can lead to discontinuing medication, only to have the illness return). As much as I know you both would like to believe this, it really is better to think of the illness as "hibernating" or as being dormant, because the tendency for someone with bipolar disorder to have additional episodes does not disappear. *Once you have bipolar disorder, you always have bipolar disorder, no matter how long you go without having a mood episode.*

One Factor That Increases Cycling: Age

Another unfortunate reality of bipolar illness is that the length of time between episodes tends to decrease as people get older. This has been found to be true for both types of bipolar disorder (I and II). I know this is not something you want to hear, and I myself had a hard time with this fact. My husband, on the other hand, who is a perpetual optimist, pointed out to me, and rightly so, that I've done a lot better during the later years of my illness, during the period that I got treatment and made important lifestyle changes, than during the earlier years.

I also think it's important to remember that when studies report findings like this they are based on *averages* of groups of people, not on individual results. And, as is true for almost everything that has to do with the course of bipolar disorder, what happens to people with this illness varies quite markedly from one person to another.

However, if you are reading this at a time where you're seeing that your partner's episodes are coming closer and closer together, I'm sure you're very concerned and want to know what, if anything, you or your mate can do to reduce the cycling. The first thing, of course, if your partner is under the care of a physician, is to consult the doctor to see if a change in medication is in order. The second thing would be to look for physical and/or psychological triggers that may be precipitating the mood episodes, and for the two of you to work together on reducing their presence when that's possible. I'll be talking about stressors briefly later on in this chapter and in more depth in Chapter 7. Suffice it to say for now that once you know what is likely to set your partner "off," you may be able to play a role in helping to stop a spark from becoming a fire.

Bipolar Triggers and Kindling Theory

Some experts believe that the reason episodes come more frequently as one ages is that they are more easily triggered or require less of a trigger (or require no trigger at all) as the number of them increases. This explanation is consistent with "kindling theory," which refers to the ability of a mental illness to take on a life of its own. It's hypothesized that while the first episode of illness may occur in response to a major stressor—like losing a job or going through a bad breakup— subsequent episodes are triggered by increasingly less stressful events. Ultimately, the illness develops the ability to set itself off (like kindling), so that very minimal or even no stressors are needed to initiate new episodes of illness. (My own personal belief is that there is always some type of trigger that precipitates mood episodes. Such triggers may seem minimal or not look at all like stressors to others, so that they go unrecognized, or they may be thoughts or hormonal shifts—see page 51—which obviously can't be witnessed by an observer.)

Dealing with Recurrence

How do you deal with the knowledge (and the anxiety that comes from knowing) that the illness is likely to come back? In order to have something akin to a normal life I think it's very important to adopt the outlook of "being here now." What I mean by this is that you try very hard to live life in the present moment and not look too far into the future.

A good example of being in the now for me is the act of writing this book. As I'm doing this right now I'm totally focused on (and enjoying) the process of writing. I'm not thinking about getting this chapter done (or the whole book either, for that matter). All of my attention is riveted on what I'm trying to communicate at this moment. As a result, *right now* I'm completely relaxed, not at all stressed.

This approach to life has the flavor of an Eastern philosophy. (And, actually, you or your mate or the two of you may find that meditation practices help in developing this mindset; see the Resources section for recommended reading.) The American way usually is to keep your eye on the goal, not focusing so much on the process of getting there as much as on gaining the prize. While certainly it's important for all of us to have goals and look forward to achieving them, I encourage you to entertain the idea that you and your loved one might benefit from paying somewhat more attention to the "now" than perhaps you're used to doing. By doing so you both will greatly reduce your anxiety about the future, which will help to normalize your present.

But what if you do need to plan ahead for something? For instance, say the two of you want to take a trip. Well, in a situation like this I usually suggest to my patients and their significant others that they try to schedule the vacation no more than a few weeks in advance, just to be on the safe side (assuming, of course, that they are doing well at the present time). This generally cuts back on the anxiety that comes from anticipating whether or not the bipolar person will be okay at that later point in time.

I know that it may not be feasible to take this suggestion in all cases. If your job requires that you request vacation time far in advance, or the place you want to go necessitates your booking reservations early (such as if you want to use your frequent flyer miles), you won't be able to be quite so flexible. But if you can minimize the time between deciding to do something and the date when you will be doing it, I recommend that you do so.

How Long Do Mood Episodes Last?

Like frequency, the length of time that mood episodes persist is highly variable among individuals—lasting for days, weeks, months, or even, for some people, years. For each individual, though, episode length tends to be relatively consistent.

Untreated Mood Episodes

Studies conducted before the availability of medication for bipolar disorder suggest that on average untreated mood episodes (of any type) go on for about 6 months. Looking at specific types of mood episodes, we know that manic and hypomanic episodes tend to be shorter—lasting days, weeks, or a few months—than major depressive episodes, which frequently go on for many months or, in some cases, for a year or more.

Research indicates that bipolar II depressions persist for longer periods of time than bipolar I depressions, nearly twice as long (1 year versus 6 months). Also, for both forms of the illness, but particularly strikingly for bipolar II disorder, the total percentage of time people are depressed is much higher than the total percentage of time they are manic or hypomanic (ratios are 3:1 and 37:1 for bipolar I and II, respectively). So if your loved one has bipolar II disorder, it's likely that most of the time he will be fighting depression, not hypomania.

Mixed episodes of bipolar illness, where both mania and depression exist concurrently, generally last for weeks to several months, but about one-third of people still have significant symptoms of the mood disturbance 1 year after it has started. And it's not unusual for a mixed episode to change into a major depressive episode or, less frequently, a manic one.

The Manic–Depression "Switch"

Over half of bipolar individuals go directly from one episode of mood disorder to another without having an intervening period of normal mood. The order of the "switch"—mania (or mixed episode or hypomania) to depression or depression to mania (or mixed episode or hypomania)—tends to be the same for a given person. For example, I have the hypomanic-to-depressed pattern—my highs occur first and then are immediately followed by lows. (That's one of the reasons I take my medication so religiously—the ups were never worth the downs that inevitably followed.)

Substance Abuse Lengthens Episodes

As I explain later in this chapter, and again in other chapters further on in this book, as mood episodes develop many people abuse alcohol or prescription medications or use street drugs, all of which can lengthen (as well as worsen) episodes.

The good news is that with the treatments that are available today—for both mood disorder and substance abuse—there really is no reason why anyone, including your partner, should have to suffer through months of distress. As you'll learn, there are many very effective medications that work in relatively brief periods of time, as well as several types of psychological therapies that have been shown to reduce the duration of mood episodes.

How Do You React to Your Partner during an Episode?

Many of the family members whom I interact with tell me they feel like they have to be with their ill partners during mood episodes almost all the time to make sure everything's okay. While I understand this sentiment, it certainly is not good for your own mental health to keep a constant vigil over your loved one (see Chapter 10 for a discussion on taking care of you). Although there is a role for you to play in helping your significant other with his mental health, ultimately your partner (and his doctor) is responsible for taking care of his emotional state.

Also, it doesn't really do much good for your significant other or your relationship for you to be hovering over your loved one nonstop. If your mate is having a depressive episode, your doting may make her feel like more of a burden than she already feels, or reinforce feelings of helplessness and inadequacy. If your loved one is hypomanic or manic, she may feel like you are "being controlling" and/or getting in the way of what she wants to do, and she may become angry and resentful.

When to be there and when to back off? How to help without being too invasive or intrusive or completely depleting yourself so you no longer are of help to your mate or yourself? I'll be going into this at length later in this book.

Four Facts You and Your Partner Need to Know

- Bipolar disorder is a chronic, recurrent illness that, at present, has no cure.
- Even though a person can go for a long period of time without signs of the illness, the propensity to have mood episodes does not go away.
- Medication is essential to preventing new episodes of illness (more on the importance of medication in Chapters 4 and 6).
- Stress often contributes to recurrence; therefore, reducing stress and mitigating its impact (when it's unavoidable) are important to mood stability; see Chapter 7.

How Will My Partner Be in between Episodes?

What does it mean to be between episodes? Will your partner return completely to normal? Will you feel like you have to walk around on tiptoe to avoid triggering another episode? How will your loved one feel and function? Let's look at some answers to these questions.

Complete versus Partial Recovery

Some people (some studies suggest most people, while others yield percentages of only 25 to 35%) have a *complete recovery* following a mood episode. A complete recovery is the same as having the disorder "in remission." This means your partner will be relatively free of mood symptoms and able to function at the level he was at prior to the mood episode—not better and not worse. This is often referred to as "a return to baseline."

Other people have only a *partial recovery* after a mood episode. If this is true for your mate, she will no longer meet the full criteria for a mood episode, but will continue to have some symptoms that are distressing, and/or the ability to function at work or in a social capacity will still be impaired in some way.

A partial recovery is more common for episodes of illness that include mood-incongruent psychotic features; that is, delusions or hallucinations that do not revolve around depressive or manic "themes." An example of this is your mate believing that her thoughts are being broadcast to others or that people can read her mind.

The fact that people with bipolar II do not, by definition, have psychotic features during their highs, and are less likely than people who have bipolar I to have them during depressions, suggests that they have a greater chance of complete remission in between mood episodes. For the most part in my practice I've found this to be true, and in my own case I've been fortunate to experience this.

Double Depression

If your mate has had a partial remission following an episode of major depression, it's likely that a similar pattern will emerge after future episodes. Sometimes this is due to the existence of a "double depression." Individuals who have double depression—periods of mild depression (dysthymia) in addition to more severe episodes of depression that qualify for a diagnosis of major depression—can be expected to have some symptoms of depression remaining after passing through an episode of major depression. For them, a return to pre-episode functioning means returning to a state of dysthymia.

Partial Recovery Leading to Complete Recovery

Some people go through a period of partial recovery that eventually leads to complete recovery. In the short term this can mean taking time off from one's job and/or gradually reentering the workplace. That's what happened to Mary Ann.

Mary Ann was a full-time professor at a small liberal arts college. She had her first manic episode at age 28, for which she was hospitalized. After being stabilized and released from the hospital, she found she couldn't return to work full-time, that the stress of teaching four courses a week was too much for her. With the dean's approval she reduced her course load to two classes for the spring semester. By the time fall rolled around she was doing much better and was able to go back to her old schedule.

He's in Remission, but Will He Be Able to Reconnect with Others?

People can find it difficult to reconnect with others even though they may be in a period of remission. They may be embarrassed by the behavior they displayed during a mood episode or may not know how to explain their seeming "absence," or they may be afraid to get involved with people again because they fear having another episode. Sometimes too much time has passed to recapture what was once there. That's what happened to Katie and Matt.

During her last episode of major depression Katie completely withdrew from all social contact, including spending time with her fiancé, Matt. When the depression ended and she felt like herself again, Katie tried to reestablish the relationship with Matt, but there had been too much damage and she wasn't able to pick up the pieces. As a result, Katie and Matt finally agreed to go their separate ways.

Please don't think that this is what has to happen to your relationship. As an example, my husband and I have been together for 22 years, and we celebrated our 20th anniversary this year. And we're not alone: many bipolar individuals and their partners successfully survive mood episodes and move forward together after they're over. Of course, reducing the probability of having additional mood episodes by taking medication and using self-help strategies that have been proven to help ward off mood swings is really your mate's best bet for ensuring her own health and the health of your union.

Deteriorating Course

Before we leave the subject of interepisode recovery, I need to tell you that a small percentage of people, unfortunately, have a progressively deteriorating course, functioning at increasingly lower levels following each mood episode.

After having three mixed episodes in 5 years, Marjorie has watched her husband, Howard, become less and less like his old self. No longer able to function in his administrative job, Howard has taken a much lesser position that, while not paying as well, has very little stress. And although once a very social person, Howard now has intense anxiety around other people, so much so that the couple's friendships have fallen by the wayside.

If you are in a situation like this, please know that I understand how very difficult this must be for you. When someone you love becomes less able to function because of any type of chronic illness, it's very sad and at the same time very stressful. You may have to take over roles your mate used to perform and give up aspects of the life you used to have together. Your dreams for the future probably will change too. That doesn't mean the two of you don't have things to look forward to. It just means you'll need to adjust your expectations, a subject I'll talk about more a little later in this book.

What Sets Off Mood Episodes?

Mood episodes can develop following a number of physical or environmental situations or stressors.

Disturbances of the Sleep–Wake Cycle

As you know from Chapter 1, decreased sleep can be a symptom of mania, hypomania, and depression, but it also can contribute to their development. In particular, it's quite common for reduced sleep to trigger mania or hypomania or to turn hypomania into mania.

After Aisha was up for several nights because of her son's illness, her mood quickly became hypomanic. Although he knew the potential consequences of cutting back on his sleep, Brent worked well into the morning hours on a special project that was due at the end of the week. His hypomanic drive quickly escalated into a manic episode. During their recent vacation, Charlie and his wife stayed out late with the other couple who came on the cruise with them. After just two nights of reduced sleep, Charlie was hypomanic.

(Because reduced sleep can elevate mood, sleep deprivation has been used as a treatment for bipolar depression. However, as you'll see in Chapter 4, it has the possibility of triggering hypomania, so it should be used only with caution and under a doctor's care.)

While insufficient sleep has consistently been implicated as a trigger of mood episodes, research also shows that *any disruption or change* of the normal sleep–wake cycle is disturbing, even if the person ends up getting his usual amount of sleep. This means that going to bed late and then "sleeping in" is not a good idea for bipolar people. It's much better to have regular, set times when one goes to bed and wakes up, preferably remaining the same on weekends as well as weekdays.

Other alterations of the usual sleep–wake cycle can be equally problematic. For instance, it's not unusual for bipolar people to have trouble when resetting their clocks for the beginning or end of daylight savings time. Changing time zones when traveling also can trigger mood episodes.

Steve loves to travel with his wife, Linda, but finds that abruptly and dramatically changing time zones can send him into a manic state. So rather than going to very faraway places, they pick vacation spots that involve only a 1- or 2-hour time change. Also, before they go on a trip, Steve gradually shifts his sleep–wake schedule over the course of a few days so that he is accustomed to the "new time" by the time he reaches his destination. For example, leaving the Midwest for a trip to New York, Steve starts moving his bedtime and wake time ahead the week before the trip, in 15-minute increments each day, until he's functioning pretty much on Eastern Standard Time.

Changes in Routine

Changes in routine other than those that affect the sleep–wake cycle also can have a major impact on the development of mood episodes. In fact, understanding the effect of this in part has formed the basis of one type of psychological therapy that has been found to be effective for bipolar individuals—interpersonal and social rhythm therapy, discussed in Chapter 4.

For many reasons, vacations are difficult for me. First of all, they usually involve a change in time zone. Even if they don't, I have difficulty sleeping in any place other than my own bedroom. Finally, there's no question that my normal day-to-day routine is completely altered when I'm away from home. But because my husband likes to travel, I've developed ways to try to get around some of these issues. Like Steve and his wife, we try to take trips that don't involve drastic time changes. We also schedule flights at times that won't interfere with my normal sleep–wake cycle (like avoiding flights that leave at 7:00 A.M. or that would have us arrive home at midnight). As for sleeping well away from home, I use all of my best "sleep hygiene" tricks (which I'll share with you in Chapter 7). And, finally, I develop for myself a vacation "routine" so that I have similar "anchor points" from one day to the next, such as getting my exercise (walking) in after breakfast each morning.

Seasonal Patterns

Some people have a seasonal pattern to their bipolar disorder. Although our psychiatric classification system acknowledges this only for episodes of depression, there have been many reports of people having a seasonal pattern to mania and hypomania as well.

The most common pattern seems to be a fall or winter depression and a spring or summer mania. (As you'll recall from Chapter 1, this is reminiscent of seasonal affective disorder, which shows a similar relationship to the seasons, at least for the fall and winter.) Most experts in this area believe that these seasonal variations in mood are caused by changes in the amount of daylight that occur at different times of the year—less daylight in fall and winter associated with depression and more daylight in the spring and summer associated with mania.

Bipolar individuals who have winter depressions—that is, they have depressions only during the winter months, or the vast majority of their depressions occur at this time of year as opposed to other times of the year—are likely to have certain characteristic symptoms during their lows. These include:

- Lack of energy
- Hypersomnia (sleeping too much)
- Carbohydrate cravings (urges to eat sweets and starches)
- Overeating with weight gain
- Reverse diurnal variation

Reverse diurnal variation means that, instead of the usual pattern seen in depressed people, with the worst mood being at the start of the day and improving as the day progresses, these individuals have their best mood when they get up in the morning and then their mood deteriorates as the day goes on.

People who have winter depressions that have this symptom profile may have a particularly good response to *phototherapy* (see Chapter 4). Phototherapy increases daily exposure to bright visual-spectrum light. (You'll remember, perhaps, from Chapter 1 that when I was living in the north I used a tanning booth to increase my light exposure. I'm convinced this helped a lot with my wintertime blues.)

If your mate has a seasonal pattern to her mood swings, you might feel like you two have little control over them—after all, you can't do anything about changes of season. But, to the contrary, in this situation forewarned is forearmed: knowing that the episode is coming allows the two of you and, if your mate is under professional care, your partner's doctors to be prepared. Together you may be able circumvent the mood episode or at least minimize its severity.

Stressful Life Events

Psychologically stressful events—like the death of someone close, a marital separation or divorce, interpersonal conflict, work-related stress, even changing residences—can precipitate the development of a mood episode. The general consensus among experts in this field is that events like these contribute more to the timing of mood episodes than to the underlying predisposition (biological–genetic) to have them.

This last stressor I just mentioned—moving—reminds me of a patient I started treating a few years ago. Although Donna had a long history of the rapid-cycling form of bipolar disorder, with medication and therapy she had been able to achieve good mood stability for nearly a year. Because she felt so well, she and her husband decided they would buy a new (bigger and better) home in another town, leaving the place where they had both grown up. Although Donna usually spoke to me about important decisions in her life, she didn't share her plans to move with me. (After the move, when I finally became aware of it, I asked her why she didn't talk to me about it. She said she knew I would think it was a bad idea [which was probably true] and she didn't want to be swayed by my opinion.)

Unfortunately, as I would have predicted for this individual, the move to the new town was disastrous to her mental health. The physical strain of the move itself (packing and unpacking, etc.), being in unfamiliar surroundings and away from her friends, and changing her everyday routine got Donna rapid cycling again. And this time she was worse than I'd ever seen her, so despondent that she was considering suicide. While she got through this crisis without inflicting harm on herself, she remained unsettled and cycling for the next year. Donna eventually realized that her new location simply wasn't going to work out for her, and, with my encouragement and support, she and her husband went back to their hometown. Thankfully, since then Donna's been doing very well.

Donna and her husband had options about where they chose to live. But what if the couple had been forced to move, say because Donna's or her husband's job required them to relocate? In that case, there are several things Donna could have done to help her make the transition to the new location. Frequent visits to the new town before the move could have reduced some of the stress associated with being in an unfamiliar place. Donna and her husband also could have joined a church or synagogue so they would have social support and structure built into their new lives. And if their moving budget had allowed, perhaps Donna could have had some help with packing and unpacking the contents of her home.

As with a job relocation, sometimes you'll be faced with stressful circumstances over which you have no control, in which case you and your partner just need to use all available resources to make a difficult situation as manageable as possible. But when faced with stressful situations over which you have some control, it's important to consider the potential stress of the life choices you make together. Minimizing stress will help maximize your mate's mood stability.

"Small" Stressors That Have a Big Impact

It's not always major life stressors, however, like the ones I mentioned at the start of this section, that trigger a mood problem. Stress is "in the eye of the beholder," and people have their own idiosyncratic triggers, some of which may seem quite minor or even silly to you but may be quite stressful to your partner. If you two know which situations these are, you'll be in a better position to avoid them or, at least, to minimize their potential impact.

For example, a situation that creates a lot of anxiety for me, which I think most other people wouldn't regard as stressful, is going to see a physician—almost any type of doctor. I know this may sound strange, particularly as I am a psychologist, and I'm not entirely sure why this is difficult for me (although I have some hunches). But because I know it's an issue, I never schedule two doctor's appointments in any given week. I spread them out so that I don't get "overloaded." I also find it helpful that my husband knows appointments with physicians are difficult for me. He almost always offers to come with me, which I appreciate even when I don't take him up on it. He also tries not to put any additional pressure on me on the days of these visits. (We'll work together to discover your mate's mood episode triggers and how to handle them when we get to Chapter 7.)

Substance-Induced Mood Episodes

Manic and depressive episodes can be triggered by prescription drugs, alcohol, or street drugs. However, some experts in this field have questioned whether these mood reactions are truly episodes of bipolar illness. Do they stem from an internal (biological–genetic) vulnerability that's then triggered by one of these substances, or are they "pseudo"-episodes of illness, brought on simply by a drug and not reflective of an underlying disease? My own personal opinion on this is that mood episodes that are precipitated by substances probably reflect a predisposition toward a mood disorder.

Substances That Trigger or Worsen Mania

The substances that most commonly induce (and also exacerbate) mania are cocaine and amphetamines, both stimulants. Prescription amphetamine derivatives and amphetamine-like substances, like Ritalin and Adderall, that frequently are used to treat attention-deficit/hyperactivity disorder, also fall into this category. Some people have developed mania-like highs from over-the-counter herbal stimulants, like ephedra, also known as *ma-huang*.

Alcohol also has been implicated as a trigger of manic episodes. However, since alcohol and stimulants often are abused during ongoing episodes of mania—stimulants to get a higher and longer high; alcohol to decrease the "raciness" that comes with mania—the substance use may be more a consequence of the mood disturbance than a cause. In either case, whether the substances are causes or consequences, there's no doubt that their use exacerbates bipolar illness.

Research has shown that antidepressant medications can trigger mania. The manic "switch rate," as it's called—the frequency with which the drugs induce mania—is different for different antidepressants. Some of these medications have rates as high as 10%, while the rate of others is near 0. Antidepressants also seem to have the ability to induce rapid cycling in bipolar people. (As you might expect, these findings for antidepressants can pose a conundrum for the psychiatrist who treats bipolar depression, an issue we'll address in Chapter 4.)

Medical Conditions That Can Mimic
or Exacerbate Bipolar Disorder

Medical conditions that are well known for triggering mania-like or depressed mood states involve the endocrine system, specifically the thyroid and the adrenal glands. Mania-like states can be caused by hyperthyroidism, a metabolism that's too fast due to an overactive thyroid gland, and Cushing's disease, a rare disorder that's caused by excessive production of cortisol by the adrenal glands or the excessive use of steroids. On the other hand, depressed mood can be due to hypothyroidism, a metabolism that's too slow due to an underactive thyroid gland (if your partner has this problem, I highly recommend the book *Thyroid Power,* by Richard and Karilee H. Shames), and Addison's disease, an uncommon condition caused by a serious reduction in the function of the adrenal glands. (While we're on the subject of hormones, I should mention that female hormonal shifts related to menstruation, giving birth, and menopause can contribute to the expression of bipolar disorder too, as I'll discuss when we get into the effects of gender on the course of bipolar disorder.)

A vitamin B_{12} deficiency has been reported to precipitate manic behavior as well as depression. Some of the other B vitamins—B_6 and folic acid—and the mineral chromium picolinate also have been linked to depression.

Hormone, vitamin, and mineral levels usually can be determined by simple blood tests, so there's no reason why any and all of the conditions above can't be checked easily by your internist or family physician. There are certain more elaborate procedures that endocrinologists use to ascertain hormone imbalances (like 24-hour urine collections and hormone "challenge" tests), so if you suspect that this may be a problem for your partner, you might encourage him or her to see a specialist.

Steroids also have been known to cause mood swings and are thought to be particularly likely to induce mania. For this reason, physicians tend to be very careful about prescribing oral cortisone and other steroids for bipolar patients. Fortunately for me, when I needed it for a back injury I did not find it affected my mood (in fact, it might have helped stabilize my mood to some extent because it eliminated a good deal of the pain I was experiencing). However, don't assume your partner's experience will be the same as mine. And, if your mate has had a problem with cortisone in the past, she's likely to have the same type of reaction in the future.

Substances That Trigger or Worsen Depression

Alcohol can precipitate or aggravate bipolar depression. People who use alcohol to try to block the painful emotions that come with their lows typically find it works for only a brief period of time. Then the depressant effect of the drug leaves them even worse off than before they started to drink.

Common prescription and over-the-counter medications that can cause or exacerbate depression include certain antihistamines, some tranquilizers, barbiturates, the acne drug Accutane, birth control pills, and certain blood pressure medications.

Is Your Partner Abusing Substances?

If your partner is abusing alcohol, prescription medications, or street drugs, he will need to be treated for this problem along with the bipolar disorder. Don't assume that substance abuse will automatically cease once your partner's bipolar disorder is under control. If anything, it's the other way around: the substance problem has to be eliminated for the bipolar disorder to be treated successfully. I'll talk about interventions for substance abuse in Chapter 7.

Does Age at the Start of the Illness Matter?

I mentioned earlier that mood episodes often occur more frequently as bipolar individuals age. But what about the beginning of the disorder? Does it matter when your partner first developed the illness? Does the age when it started affect the course of the disorder?

Research that has compared those whose bipolar disorder started in adolescence with those whose illness began in adulthood has shown no difference in the number of mood episodes experienced over time or their severity. But when looking at bipolar individuals who first developed the illness in early childhood, before puberty, the picture changes.

Findings from short-term (2-year) follow-up studies show that young children with bipolar disorder have a more severe form of bipolar disorder—a continuous, very-rapid-cycling course with primarily mixed symptoms and no recovery between episodes (since they virtually always are in an episode)—than adolescents and adults, who mostly have discrete episodes of illness that typically last for weeks or months and alternate with full or partial recovery.

The difference in outcome for young children may be due to heavier "genetic loading" for the disorder—more relatives with mood disorders and bipolar disorder in particular, sometimes with bipolar disorder appearing on both sides of the family—than in individuals who have the more typical adolescent or adult onset.

What about the long-term course of individuals who develop bipolar disorder at a very young age? Do the episodes change from chronic, very rapid cycling into the discrete episodes that are characteristic of individuals with a late adolescent or adult onset? Surprisingly, there's virtually no information on this subject, probably because the answer can require a lengthy prospective follow-up period (following children through adolescence and well into adulthood). My educated guess, though, if I had to predict, is that bipolar disorder with a childhood onset is probably associated with a more chronic course and poorer outcome, such as is true of many other major psychiatric disorders. Science, however, is not based on speculation, so we'll have to wait for findings from well-conducted research studies before we can answer this question.

Does Gender Affect Course?

The course of bipolar disorder for men and women differs in several ways. The very first episode of illness in women usually is a major depression, while it typically is mania in men. Also, on average women have twice as many depressed episodes throughout their illness than men.

Interestingly, although bipolar disorder is distributed equally between women and men, the rapid-cycling form of the illness, which is present in 5 to 15% of bipolar I and II individuals, is much more common among females (about three-quarters are women). Several theories have been proposed to account for this finding. One is that women are more likely than men to have thyroid problems, which have been found to be related to rapid-cycling. Another is that female hormones, estrogen in particular, account for the difference between men and women. Finally, it has been postulated that women may be more likely to be on antidepressant medication (because, as I said earlier, they have more depressed episodes than men) and that this may be causing the rapid-cycling.

Thirty-nine-year-old Kimberly has not been treated for her rapid-cycling bipolar disorder. For 3 weeks of every month she's depressed—crying, wringing her hands, wishing to be dead, hating herself, calling herself fat and stupid. During the 4th week of the month, she switches to hypomania—extremely cheerful but irritable and agitated if crossed, thinking she's much better than other people, very productive and full of energy but requiring less sleep.

Although, as I've suggested before, the rapid-cycling form of bipolar disorder tends to have a poorer prognosis than other forms of bipolar disorder (particularly when it's not treated), new psychiatric medications and the use of certain other agents—like the active form of thyroid hormone (T3 or cytomel)—have been shown to play a useful role in its management. So if your mate has the rapid-cycling form of bipolar illness, there's reason to be optimistic. I'll discuss this in more depth when we get to Chapter 4.

The Effects of Hormonal Changes on Bipolar Women

If your partner is female, you may be wondering how the flux of sex hormones affects the course of her illness.

"My wife is worse at certain times of the month. Is that typical of bipolar disorder?"

Since many women who do not have bipolar disorder report having symptoms of anxiety and/or depression in the days prior to menstruation (premenstrual syndrome), it would be logical to guess that bipolar symptoms would worsen in the days preceding menses. Actually the research evidence varies: in some studies a significant number of bipolar women have reported worsening of their depressive symptoms several days before menstruating; other studies have not shown this relationship. So all we can conclude at this time is that having or not having a pattern to mood episodes that's related to menstruation is a very individual issue.

"How will she be after having a baby? I've heard the postpartum period is rough for women who have bipolar disorder."

As I highlighted in the story at the very beginning of this chapter, of all the times in a bipolar woman's life, the greatest risk of having a mood episode comes after giving birth. Although the reason for this susceptibility is not entirely clear, many think it has to do with the rapid and dramatic hormone changes that occur during the postpartum period. It also may be related to the emotional and physical stress (including sleep deprivation) associated with labor, delivery, and having a newborn. For some women, postpartum changes actually trigger the onset of bipolar disorder; for others, it's a continuation of an illness that's already reared its head.

Women more commonly experience postpartum depression, but postpartum mania can occur instead (this is what usually has been referred to in the media as "postpartum psychosis"). If a manic episode develops during the postpartum period, there may be an increased risk for recurrence in subsequent postpartum periods.

The postpartum risk for mood episodes, along with a number of other factors, may affect your decision about whether to have children. I'll be talking about this very difficult and sensitive topic in more depth in Chapter 10. For now the first thing you and your significant other need to do is to make an honest appraisal of your partner's illness, specifically, the extent to which your loved one currently is ill and is likely to be so in the future. Can your partner handle all the demands of child rearing? Is your loved one in a position to devote the time and attention that an infant (or toddler, or young child) requires?

Susan has bipolar I disorder with psychotic features and has resisted taking the medication her doctor prescribed. For her and her husband, having offspring may not be a realistic option. By contrast, Georgia has a mild version of bipolar II disorder and has been well stabilized for several years. She and her partner may be able to manage having children in their lives.

Another thing to consider is what medications your partner takes and whether she can continue to take them during part or all of her pregnancy. Finally, knowing the extent to which bipolar disorder runs in your partner's family (and the type of bipolar disorder it is) can help you assess the genetic risk for the illness that may be conferred to your child.

Looking at all this, my husband and I ultimately decided not to have children. I'm sure you'll understand when I tell you that this was one of the most difficult and painful decisions we ever have had to make, as I am sure it could be for you and your partner. It also was a true test of our relationship, which you know by now has stood strong for more than two decades.

"How will my wife's bipolar disorder be during and after menopause?"

Because of the dramatic mood swings that appear to be caused by the rapidly fluctuating hormones that occur during the perimenopause and menopause periods, bipolar women can find these stages of the life cycle particularly difficult to handle. On the other hand, if your mate has had the rapid-cycling form of bipolar disorder, it's possible (at least it's been hypothesized) that the decrease in estrogen that takes place as a result of menopause could ultimately increase the length of time between mood cycles.

Emily, who is 47 and has bipolar disorder, has been having a harder time since she entered menopause. She now has times when

Women and Bipolar Disorder

- A woman's first episode of illness is likely to be a major depression.
- During the course of their illness, bipolar women have twice as many depressive episodes as bipolar men.
- Women are more likely than men to have the rapid-cycling form of bipolar disorder, by a ratio of 3:1.
- There is no clear relationship between the female monthly menstrual cycle and the timing of bipolar symptoms—it's different for different women.
- Women are at the highest risk for a mood episode after giving birth, that is, during the postpartum period.

her moods seem to vary from hour to hour. Emily is confused about whether this extreme moodiness is tied up with her changing hormones or the bipolar disorder is worse. All she knows is that she doesn't feel like her self. To get to the bottom of this, her psychiatrist suggests that she see her gynecologist or an endocrinologist to check out her hormone levels.

Male Sex Hormones and Bipolar Disorder

Before leaving the topic of gender and hormones, I think it's important to point out that many men also go through a period later in life when their sex hormones decline, similar to the female menopause (instead, it's called *andropause*). Decreasing levels of testosterone (which usually start to occur in men aged 50 and up) have been linked to depression, which, in turn, can exacerbate bipolar disorder. So if your mate is a male in this age range, he might want to consider having a simple blood test (done by his internist or an endocrinologist) to check his amount of free-circulating testosterone. Testosterone replacement therapy may be an option. (To learn more about this problem, as well as its treatment, I recommend the book *The Testosterone Syndrome* by Eugene Shippen and William Fryer.)

Will My Partner Develop Other Psychiatric Illnesses?

Does my mate's bipolar disorder predispose her to develop additional problems? Or could the bipolar disorder "turn into" another type of illness?

Schizophrenia

As I said in Chapter 1, sometimes doctors have difficulty distinguishing actively psychotic manias from schizophrenia. Perhaps that's why partners and other family members of my bipolar patients frequently ask me, particularly when the diagnosis is bipolar I with psychotic features, whether a loved one's condition could turn into schizophrenia. Let me assure you that *people who have bipolar disorder are not at increased risk of developing schizophrenia.* The doctor's obtaining a careful and complete history of the illness and following up with your partner over time can ensure that your loved one's condition is diagnosed accurately.

Personality Disorders

As I discussed in Chapter 1, it's not unusual for bipolar individuals to have personality disorders as well. But since personality disorders, *by definition,* have their onset in adolescence and are well established by early adulthood, a person who does not already have such a disorder cannot develop one later on in life.

Anxiety Disorders

Many bipolar individuals have anxiety disorders—panic disorder, social anxiety disorder, obsessive–compulsive disorder, generalized anxiety disorder, posttraumatic stress disorder, and phobias—in addition to their bipolar disorders. These disorders can precede or follow the onset of bipolar disorder, but in either event, they will be important for your mate to deal with since anxiety (in addition to being a problem in its own right) often precipitates the development of a mood episode, particularly hypomania and mania.

Substance Abuse

As I'll discuss at length in Chapter 7, bipolar individuals are at a greatly increased risk of having alcohol or drug abuse or dependence. In fact more than half (60%) do. Substance abuse can mask bipolar disorder, making it harder to diagnose. As I mentioned earlier, it also can worsen the course of the disorder by lengthening mood episodes and increasing their severity. Of greatest concern, however, as you'll see in the next section, is the fact that substance use problems among bipolar individuals are strongly associated with suicidal behavior.

Does Bipolar II Disorder Turn into Bipolar I Disorder?

Although this isn't technically an issue of developing another psychiatric disorder, if your partner has bipolar II disorder I'm sure you're wondering how likely it is that your loved one's illness will turn into bipolar I disorder, the more severe form of bipolar illness. I'm happy to let you know that very few bipolar II individuals—estimates range from 5 to 15%—ever develop true manic episodes.

Some experts believe that this finding supports the notion that bipolar I and II disorders are separate, although related, illnesses. Studies of illness in family members support this idea. While bipolar I individuals have family members with both bipolar I and II in their family trees, those with bipolar II tend to have *only* bipolar II, not bipolar I.

Mortality Risks in Bipolar Disorder

It's a sad fact that the mortality rate is twice as high for people with bipolar disorder as for people of the same age who do not have the illness. Recent data suggest that the top three causes of death for bipolar individuals, in their order of frequency, are cardiovascular disease, suicide, and accidents.

Cardiovascular Disease

One risk factor for heart disease that is potentially modifiable is smoking. Rather alarmingly, several studies have shown that 55% of those with bipolar disorder smoke cigarettes. As troubling as this figure is, I don't find it surprising. Nicotine is a biphasic drug—it can both stimulate and, alternatively, relax people, depending on the dose (how many cigarettes are smoked). Because of these effects, I believe, many people struggling with bipolar symptoms use cigarettes as a mood stabilizer.

I know that when I quit smoking 10 years ago I became much more emotionally labile—that is, my mood was more easily changeable—than ever before. I would cry more easily and get angry more easily, and this went on for several years, so it wasn't just a withdrawal symptom. Finally, when my medication was adjusted, the problem stopped.

Another cardiovascular risk factor is the presence of the *metabolic syndrome*. The metabolic syndrome is defined as having three or more of the following five conditions:

- Abdominal obesity—defined as a waist circumference of greater than 40 inches in men and 35 inches in women
- Elevated triglycerides
- Elevated cholesterol
- High blood pressure
- High fasting blood glucose levels

Unfortunately, several medications that are very effective for bipolar illness have been shown to increase the likelihood of developing the metabolic syndrome, particularly when taken at higher doses. (As with the treatment of any illness, the risks of the treatment, or potential adverse effects, need to be considered relative to the potential benefits that may be gained.) But, as I'll talk about in detail in Chapter 4, two drugs have been developed relatively recently that may be as effective in treating bipolar symptoms as their older counterparts, without increasing the risk of metabolic syndrome. As a result, many psychiatrists are switching their bipolar patients to these newer medications.

Suicide

Tragically, many of the deaths that make up the increased mortality in bipolar disorder can be attributed to suicide. Studies show that the rate of suicide deaths in bipolar I and II individuals is 10 to 15% and that about 25%, at one time or another, make an attempt on their own lives.

I know that these are tough facts to handle. No one wants to think that someone he or she loves might intentionally try to hurt himself. The important thing to keep in mind, though, is how critical prevention is to the continued safety of your partner. Mood episode prevention *is* suicide prevention.

You also should know that ***in almost half of bipolar suicides alcoholism or drug abuse is present as well as the mood disorder.*** In addition to concurrent substance abuse, suicide risk is especially high for individuals with psychotic features, a history of previous suicide attempts, and/or a family history of suicide.

Although, thankfully, I've never had a patient attempt suicide (at least that I know of, that is, while a patient was in treatment with me),

I've heard about more attempts than I care to recall. And one of the scariest aspects of such attempts is that people often use their own medication, something that's readily available to them, which in sufficient quantity can be lethal. That's why if your loved one is suicidal, certain safeguards need to be put into place so that the risk of self-harm is eliminated. This may mean your monitoring your partner's medication or requiring that your mate have a hospital stay. I'll discuss these issues more in depth in Chapters 8 and 9.

For reasons that are not entirely clear, recent data suggest that individuals with metabolic syndrome who meet the obesity criterion are more likely to report a history of suicide attempts. It may be that this finding is an artifact of illness severity—that is, that more severely ill persons (those who are likely to attempt suicide) are taking more medication (which increases the probability of obesity) and, as a result, are at increased risk for medication-induced metabolic syndrome.

Accidents

Manic delusions—like grandiose delusions, delusions of invincibility, and delusions of having special powers—can lead people to do things that can cause them harm even though they may not intentionally be trying to hurt themselves. Carrie, who has refused to be treated for her bipolar disorder, believes she's invincible. She wants to show her husband that nothing can hurt her. To prove her point she lies down in the middle of the street with traffic coming toward her. Arnold, who has stopped taking his medication, believes he can fly. He climbs onto his roof to give it a try, but is thwarted by his wife, who is able to talk him back down in the nick of time.

I know that examples like these are scary. But please keep in mind that these are people who have a severe form (the type that has psychotic features) of bipolar I disorder that is not, obviously, medically under control.

One could speculate that the high rate of accidental deaths that occur among bipolar people also is at least partially the result of the impulsivity and lack of judgment associated with manic (or mixed) episodes. For example, James, who is in a manic episode, has been in four automobile accidents in the past 2 months. He's so busy talking to people on his cell phone and distracted by things he sees around him that he's not paying proper attention to his driving. His wife worries about his continuing to be on the road—that he'll end up hurt or even worse. Finally, after an all-out screaming fight, she's taken the car keys away from him and is chauffeuring him to where he needs to go.

Battles over control when your partner is out of control are inevitable if your mate has severe episodes of mood disturbance. Although, in the short run, the arguments will cause a rift in your relationship, taking charge may literally mean saving your loved one's life.

The Benefits of Bipolar Disorder: Creativity and Leadership

Much has been written on the relationship between creativity and bipolar illness and the seemingly large number of very accomplished writers, painters, and musicians who have had the disorder. Actually, research studies have shown that this perception is supported by fact: astonishingly, 30 to 50% of successful artists suffer from bipolar illness, a prevalence rate that's at least 10 times that in the general population.

Why is this so? It probably most directly is due to changes in thought processes that are experienced during manic or hypomanic episodes. Ideas that are loosely connected and flow without inhibition can easily give rise to novel means of expression. In addition, other characteristics of manic and hypomanic states—like increased energy, drive, and productivity, the ability to take risks (calculated ones that may lead to rewards), and a heightened sense of self-confidence—also may lead creative people to turn out works of greatness.

The question arises, then, whether the treatment of bipolar disorder impairs creativity and dampens artistic expression. Actually, several studies were conducted to address this issue after lithium first became available. Contrary to expectation, results showed that over half of the artists surveyed reported that treatment with the drug actually *increased* their artistic productivity. There also was one-quarter who felt that lithium had no impact on their work, and another quarter who thought the drug had a negative influence on their work.

In addition to writers, musicians, and painters, there are bipolar people who have been hugely successful leaders in other fields, such as politics, business, and science. People like this use their hypomanic and manic periods to "go for the gold." They think and act "outside the box," which can yield tremendous rewards that further not only their own lives but also societies at large. If one thinks in terms of there being an upside to having bipolar disorder, there's no question that this most certainly is it.

I know that in my own life my hypomanic periods generally affected my work in a positive way. The ability to see things clearly and to put ideas together in imaginative ways, paired with increased drive and productivity, was my recipe for success in all aspects of my career. Can I still do my work just as well without the highs, now that my mood is stabilized on medication? I believe so, and in some ways I think even better. I may not be as fast at doing things as I used to be (I guess this could be due to getting older as well as the medication), but I believe my work is more consistent (more consistently good) than when I had highs and lows.

As you've seen in this chapter, bipolar disorder is a serious, chronic illness that, for the best outcome, requires medical treatment. But what if your partner refuses to accept that he has the illness? What if you can't get your mate to admit there's something wrong and agree to go see a doctor? The next chapter will show you what you can do to overcome the denial.

3

"It's Not Me!"

When Your Partner Is in Denial

Sharon's husband, Marty, suffers from mood swings. When he's down, he completely withdraws from her and the world, so despondent it's painful for Sharon to see. When he's up, he goes from super-cheerful to irritable and argumentative in seconds and is nasty to his wife to a point that brings her to tears.

Marty is from the "old school"—he believes people should solve their own problems and not seek help from outsiders. But after pleading with him for months Sharon finally persuaded him to see a psychiatrist for an evaluation. The doctor came up with a diagnosis—bipolar disorder—and recommended Marty try a mood-stabilizing medication. But Marty refuses to believe he is, what he calls, a manic–depressive. "I'm not crazy," he insists, "and that doctor doesn't know what he's talking about!" He won't go back to see him—or take the medication—no matter what Sharon says.

Sharon feels frustrated and helpless. She can't see them continuing to go on this way. Is there anything she can do to get Marty to accept the diagnosis and try the medication? Why won't he at least give it a chance?

As you've seen in the first two chapters of this book, bipolar disorder is a very serious, chronic, and potentially disabling illness that requires medical treatment. But what do you do if, like Sharon's husband, your partner has received the diagnosis but refuses to believe it's true? Or what if you haven't even been able to get your loved one to see a doctor because your mate won't admit anything's wrong? Whichever is the case, you're up against the same problem: *denial.*

Denial is something that bipolar people and their partners frequently have to deal with, and not just before and immediately following a diagnosis. Denial can reappear at any point during the course of the illness, even after your loved one seems to have accepted the diagnosis.

In this chapter I'll be talking mostly about the denial that occurs after your partner first receives the bipolar diagnosis. This is the type of denial that, as for Marty, is often a major stumbling block to getting treatment. But if your partner hasn't been diagnosed yet, either because he hasn't gone to see a doctor or the diagnosis hasn't been firmed up, you can still use much of what's in this chapter; the forms denial takes and the solutions to overcoming it are in many cases the same prediagnosis as postdiagnosis.

I know quite a lot about the process of denying this illness, and not just from my work with bipolar individuals and their families. Although I've had the disorder most of my life, I didn't allow myself to see it until I was past 40.

It's probably hard for you to fathom how a psychologist trained in diagnosing and treating this illness was able to close her eyes to her own situation for so many years. The only way I can explain it is to say that I honestly did not see (or did not want to see) all the evidence that was right in front of me. Despite the irrefutable facts that bipolar disorder runs in my family and that I had had clear episodes of hypomania and depression since adolescence, I was able to disassociate myself entirely from the illness.

It's not that I didn't know something was wrong. I knew I had down periods. But I attributed them to the weather (when I lived in the north), to stressful situations, and even to my physical health (I remember one time in particular when I thought I might have had mononucleosis because of how lethargic I felt). And like many other bipolar people, I thought of my up times, my happy times, as my normal self—I did not consider them a problem.

It wasn't until I hit a really bad low in my early 30s that I started thinking maybe I could benefit from medication and finally went to see a psychiatrist. The doctor told me that what I had was bipolar disorder, but I completely dismissed what she—and my own very tiny inner voice—said.

It ended up taking many more years for me to recognize—that is, truly believe—that what my doctor had told me was true. A number of small but very important steps along the way ultimately led to this awareness, many using the resources and techniques I've included in this chapter. But in the final analysis it seemed like everything came together for me in a matter of seconds—like a lightbulb lit up in my head. With extraordinary clarity at that moment I realized that I was one of these people I had been treating—that I, in fact, had bipolar disorder. I even remember saying to my psychiatrist rather incredulously, "I have bipolar disorder?" and her responding with a look of amusement on her face—for she had told me this so many times in the past—"Yes."

With this acceptance came a whole new beginning. Treatment options were open to me that I never before considered, ones that really work for this disorder. I also started to use the self-help strategies and make the lifestyle changes that I had always encouraged my bipolar patients to use. I became steadfastly determined that although I might not be able to slay this beast I would at least keep it at bay. And that's exactly what I've done. I've stopped suffering and started living.

Like me, once your loved one recognizes the illness, she can go on to have much better tomorrows. I certainly hope this happens for your mate sooner than it did for me, and my sharing my story with you and writing this book is directed toward that end. The very first step in this process, though, involves acknowledging that there is a problem and that the problem goes by the name of bipolar disorder. This means breaking through your partner's wall of denial.

I know that some of you reading this have tried many times in the past to get your partners to see that they need help but haven't yet been successful. You may feel that no matter how hard you try, you're not going to get your mate to acknowledge what's really going on, and you are exhausted and frustrated that you're not getting anywhere. But please don't give up! I'll help you see why your partner is so resistant to accepting the diagnosis and going for treatment and give you concrete suggestions to get past this, strategies that have worked for countless numbers of my patients and their families, ones that should work for you and your mate, too.

Why Your Partner Rejects the Diagnosis

People have trouble accepting that they have bipolar disorder for a number of different reasons. But the most common one, in my experience, stems from how they perceive the illness.

Nobody Wants to Be Labeled "Crazy"

The terms *bipolar* and *manic–depressive* can conjure up frightening images, many of which come from the way the classic form of the illness has been described in the medical literature and also the way it's been depicted in films and works of fiction.

In fact, the first patient I ever had contact with during my graduate school days fit this profile. When I met her, she had just been hospitalized for a psychotic mania and hadn't yet been stabilized on medication. Her anger (which really was rage) was intense and out of control—she spewed horrible comments and spit on me while I was interviewing her. (Being young and completely inexperienced, I was so deeply disturbed by this patient that I began to question whether I had gone into the right field—whether I really was cut out to be a psychologist!)

Nobody wants to think of him- or herself even remotely in this way. Fortunately, today the picture of this illness has changed. We now know bipolar disorder doesn't come only in "black and white," with psychotic manias and suicidal depressions, but also appears in "shades of gray," with variations that are much milder. Yet people still have a fear of this disorder—and there's a stigma too—that doesn't exist for many other psychiatric illnesses.

What does this mean for you and your partner? It means that if your loved one thinks of bipolar disorder in an extreme, stereotypical way, she most probably will have tremendous difficulty accepting the diagnosis. In this case, to get past this problem, your mate needs to become educated about the illness and the many different ways it can manifest itself.

A number of books in print contain personal accounts of people's journeys with bipolar disorder. If your mate can relate to one of these individuals' experiences, she might be able to accept that she too has the illness.

I know this helped me. Shortly after I was first diagnosed I read the book *Call Me Anna* by Patty Duke. I saw some of myself in her portrayal of her own illness. By contrast, I couldn't identify with Kay Redfield Jamison's book *An Unquiet Mind* (although a wonderful work of nonfiction), where she chronicles her psychotic episodes and suicide attempts. Which personal accounts your partner can identify with will depend on the nature of your partner's illness (see the Resources for a broader selection of such books you both might wish to read).

There also are a number of good books about bipolar disorder in general (some of which are particularly user-friendly, like *The Bipolar Disorder Survival Guide* by David J. Miklowitz) that provide information on different aspects of the disorder. The Internet is another excellent means of learning about bipolar disorder, and, of course, it's free. Chat rooms are useful too in making your loved one more knowledgeable about the illness—conversing with people who have problems similar to the ones your partner has can be tremendously helpful. (See the Resources at the end of this book for specific recommendations of books and Internet sources.)

But what do you do if your partner won't read the books you've brought home or the articles you've printed out from the Internet or, worse yet, gets angry at you for even suggesting that he really does have bipolar disorder? My answer is to try again at another time, a time when your mate may be more receptive, and to make sure you approach the subject in a casual way, possibly even suggesting that you look at the materials together. If this doesn't work, it still will be helpful for you to learn more about the disorder yourself. In sharing with your mate what you've discovered, you very well could start dispelling the distorted picture of the illness your partner is carrying in his head.

Nobody Wants to Take Psychiatric Medication

Most people know that having bipolar disorder means having to take medication (and anyone who doesn't already know it will know it after seeing a doctor and being diagnosed with the illness), and many have concerns or fears about this that can stop them from accepting their diagnosis and undergoing treatment. (Marty, as you'll recall from the beginning of this chapter, refused to take the mood stabilizer his doctor prescribed.)

In fact, just recently a patient of mine who has mood swings asked me, with a worried look, if I thought she had bipolar disorder. Before I answered the question, I asked her what her concern about that would be. She immediately replied in a hushed but forceful voice, "You have to take medication for that!"

There's no denying that what my patient said is true. And the medication one must take generally is for the long term, which means always, for the rest of one's life.

Why might your partner, like my patient, have trouble with the idea of taking psychiatric medication? Your mate may be concerned that psychotropic drugs alter brain chemistry (which they do) or worried that they will produce unpleasant side effects or affect her physical health. Your partner may be anxious that people will find out she is taking a psychiatric drug, that her "weakness" would be exposed. And then there's the fact that taking medication really is an acknowledgment that something is wrong with you, that you do indeed have an illness.

There are a couple of things you can do to try to get your loved one past rejecting the bipolar diagnosis because it means having to take medication. If your partner is concerned about how he is going to feel on the drug, you can approach taking the medication as an "experiment," that is, suggesting that your mate try the medication for a limited time period and then, at the end of the period, deciding whether to continue it. That's how George approached the situation with his wife, Beverly.

George: Sweetie, I know you really are frightened about taking medication.

Beverly: I don't want to be a "zombie."

George: But honey, what if the medication makes you feel better?

Beverly: But I've heard about the stuff the doctor wants me to take. It's strong. I don't know how I'll be when I'm on it.

George: You could try it over the weekend just to see how it affects you. Then, if you're okay with it, you could give it a couple of weeks and see how you feel about it then.

Beverly: I guess I could do that. I mean just try it for a couple of weeks. That would be okay.

Your loved one can become more informed about the medication that's being considered—how it works, potential short- and long-term side effects—through your partner's doctor, and/or you and your mate can turn to the resources I recommended earlier.

If your partner's primary concern is embarrassment over taking psychiatric medication, you can point out that people are taking these drugs in record numbers today so that the stigma once associated with this form of treatment really no longer exists. Moreover, with the exception of you, the doctor, and the pharmacist who fills the prescription, there's no reason anyone needs to know about your mate's treatment. It's completely up to your partner whether or not to share this information with anyone else.

Nobody Wants to Have a Chronic Illness That Has No Cure

Unlike a number of other psychiatric disorders, bipolar disorder is an illness that gets "managed," not cured. In this way it's like many other chronic medical conditions, such as diabetes or lupus.

Although it certainly is true that bipolar disorder is a chronic illness, it comes in the form of episodes, as you know if you read Chapter 2. Some people are fortunate to have many years, even decades, without mood episodes, and this is one potential positive aspect of this illness. Moreover, many people have a full or at least partial recovery between episodes, enabling them to live relatively normal lives.

The other good news is that highly effective treatments for bipolar disorder are emerging all the time. So there's reason to be quite hopeful that in your significant other's lifetime even more efficacious interventions will become available. And with all the research that's being conducted on the causes of bipolar disorder, there's always the possibility that a cure is right around the corner.

All that being said, however, it is very hard for many people to accept that they have a serious illness that is not entirely going to "go

away." If you suspect this is part of the reason your loved one continues to deny having the illness, you should try your best to approach
the situation with all the sympathy you can muster and point to the
best-case scenarios I just outlined:

- Long periods, for many, between episodes
- Good interepisode recovery
- The current and future availability of pharmacological—as well
  as psychological—treatments that really work
- The hope of a cure down the road

I can tell you from both my personal and professional experience
that optimism and hope play important roles not only in accepting this
illness but also in positively affecting its course.

Instead, or in addition, it may be that your loved one feels shame
at the idea that he or she has a *mental* illness and, possibly, is to blame
for being in this situation. Feelings like these can further distance your
mate from acceptance of the illness. If feelings of shame are the problem, you might want to point out that there are a great many very
accomplished individuals who have come forth with and shared their
own psychiatric conditions with the public (you might name a few
who've told their stories to the media) and that—as for these people—
there really is nothing to be embarrassed about. You also might make
a remark about the millions who apparently are taking medication for
mental disorders by saying something like "Look at all those com-
mercials on TV—the drug companies wouldn't be spending all that
money on them if there weren't tons of people taking those drugs." If
your mate tends toward self-recrimination, you might say something
reassuring like "Hey, you know, it's not your fault that you have this
illness—you probably inherited it," to help lessen your partner's tendencies to self-blame.

Nobody Wants to Be Unsure of Who He Really Is

Most people view their emotional reactions as originating from their
personalities, certainly not as part of a disease process. Being diagnosed with bipolar disorder, though, brings up many questions about
one's identity. Recognizing that I had the disorder forced me to consider whether my feelings, at times, were reflections of my true self or

manifestations of the illness. I wondered, "Who is the real me?" and "Where does the illness stop and I begin?" As you can imagine, questions like these can be very disturbing.

If your partner is saying things like this, you might try asking your mate to list some attributes that she thinks describe her personality—traits that are enduring regardless of the presence (or absence) of mood episodes. Chances are your loved one will be able to come up with at least a few characteristics, but if she is having problems with this, you can jump in and share traits that you see as stable, consistent personality features.

When Beth asked her fiancé, Julian, to do this, he came up with this list:

- Intelligent
- Compassionate
- Creative
- Sensitive
- Hardworking
- Honest

Doing this exercise helped Julian see that there is an "I"—a true identity—that persists despite the illness, that he has characteristics that don't go away even in the face of his mood swings.

How Your Partner Rejects the Diagnosis: The Many Faces of Denial

People with bipolar disorder manifest denial in a lot of different ways. Your partner won't necessarily come right out and say, "I don't have bipolar disorder, and therefore I don't plan to do anything about it." Your mate may try on various explanations for the mood shifts and erratic behavior, from calling them normal to blaming the world. Or denial may come in more subtle forms that could prevent your partner from taking full advantage of available interventions. Some people with bipolar disorder express their denial in different ways at different points in their lives.

Although it may be beyond your power to get your loved one to fully accept the bipolar diagnosis, if you know what denial looks like in its many forms, you can at least be prepared to nudge your mate in the right direction.

"There's Nothing Wrong with Me"

Harold has periods when he totally shuts down, taking time off from work, withdrawing from family and friends, flying, as he calls it, "under the radar." Then there are the other times, the periods when he's revved up and ready to go—planning trips to faraway places, calling people he hasn't spoken to in years, staying up late and getting up early and, as he puts it, "not wanting to miss a thing."

Karen is afraid to talk to Harold about seeing a doctor for his mood swings because the last time she brought it up he stormed out of the house and didn't come back until the next day. "What are you talking about?" he shouted. "There's nothing wrong with me!" he yelled as he slammed the door behind him.

At a loss for what to do, Karen decided to speak to their family physician on her own. The doctor said he suspected Harold might have a mild form of bipolar disorder, and, after reading up on it, Karen thinks he's probably right.

Like Harold, your mate may have great difficulty seeing that his or her moods are extreme and signs of an illness. This may be hard for you to understand because it's so apparent to you that something is wrong. But from your partner's perspective he or she may think, "This is just who I am" or "My mother was this way too," trying to normalize what you know is abnormal. In fact, this is one reason many people with bipolar disorder don't go to see a doctor, because they're convinced (or have convinced themselves) that nothing—at least nothing serious—is wrong with them. (I recently asked a relative of mine who has bipolar disorder but doesn't know it—he's never been diagnosed—how he would go about getting someone who has mood swings to see a doctor. His response, which I think is very telling, was, "Why would anyone go to a doctor for mood swings?")

> "I'm just emotional."
> "I'm moody."
> "It's my personality."
> "I've always been this way."

Karen has a difficult dilemma before her. She knows her husband has a problem and needs to get treatment, but he responds with hostility to her attempts to address it. She's worried that bringing it up again will exacerbate his anger or, even worse, that he might leave her and their three children. She feels caught between the proverbial rock and a hard place—in trouble if she doesn't do anything, because Harold's illness will continue to go untreated, and in trouble if she does, because she might make a bad situation even worse.

Is there a way for Karen to approach the issue that her husband will accept? How can you persuade someone to get help when the response you get is anger?

In raising the possibility that something may be wrong, the first thing Karen should do is to *look for the right opportunity*. Unfortunately, the last time she brought up the idea of getting help, Harold was in an angry, agitated state, so she got an angry, agitated response. Had she approached the subject at another time, a time when he was in a more level place, she may have had more success.

Another strategy that often is effective is to bring the topic up when your spouse is in a down period. When people are very low, experiencing the emotional pain of depression, they're typically more open to hearing the kind of message Karen has to deliver—that Harold really needs outside help.

A somewhat different tack Karen could have taken would be to *plant seeds* periodically; that is, at the right time, in a nonthreatening way, show Harold specific instances when his reactions to things were too intense or greater than the situation warranted. Let's take a look at an example.

Harold and Karen go out to dinner to a trendy new restaurant that doesn't take reservations. When they arrive, they are told the wait is 30 minutes. Thirty minutes pass and Harold approaches the hostess, pointing out that she had said the table would be ready by now. The hostess tells him it's taking longer than expected, that's she's terribly sorry but there's nothing she can do. Harold raises his voice loud enough for the other people waiting to hear and says, "What are you, stupid? Can't you tell time?" and rushes past Karen and out the door.

Karen says nothing outside the restaurant or in the car while Harold is speeding his way back home. She even keeps quiet about the incident during the rest of the evening while Harold continues to go on about "what a moron" the hostess was and how he's never going back to that restaurant where people think they are better than him.

The next day, when it's clear that Harold is past what happened the night before, Karen says to him: "Honey, don't you think you over-reacted somewhat to that hostess last night?" and then, since he seems to handle this comment okay, she goes on to say, "Isn't that the same type of reaction you had last week when that bank teller wasn't going fast enough for you?"

What Karen has done here is to plant two seeds. The first seed is that Harold's reaction to the hostess wasn't normal (although, of course, she doesn't use the word *normal,* or *abnormal* either, for that matter), that it was excessive—bigger than it should have been, given the situation. The second seed she plants links the situation from the previous evening with another recent incident when she observed the same behavior—a similar overreaction, but in that case to a teller at their bank.

Planting new seeds like this and "watering" those you've already planted—with soft reminders—needs to be an ongoing process. I'm not suggesting, though, that you bring up situations every day. You don't want to come across like you are nagging or nitpicking every-thing your mate does or says. If you do, your partner probably will either ignore you or become very angry, neither of which is a response you're looking for.

When your partner tries to normalize the abnormal ...

- *Communicate your partner's need for help when the mood is right*—chances are he or she will be more receptive to your message when calm or experiencing the emotional pain of depression.

- *Avoid using words and expressions that are likely to inflame your mate*—like *abnormal, sick, mental illness,* and even *bipolar disorder.*

- *Look for opportunities to plant seeds,* that is, to point out specific situations where your partner overreacted or acted inappropriately, such as the day after an incident has occurred.

- *Repeat your message* (water the seeds) periodically, but don't do it so often that you end up alienating or antagonizing your mate.

"It's Not Me; It's Everyone and Everything Else"

It's very common for bipolar people to attribute their mood swings to situations or other people, externalizing blame for how they feel rather than accepting that the problem really lies within themselves. Externalizing blame can go hand in hand with normalizing the abnormal, as in Harold's case when he blamed the hostess and the bank teller for his over-the-top anger.

It's not only small situations where your partner may point to outside events as the cause of his or her emotional reactions. Your partner may think, "If only I hadn't taken this job" or "If only I didn't live in this place" or "If only I wasn't in this relationship, I would be fine." You'll remember from the beginning of this chapter how I deflected my mood problem in this way for many years.

If your mate externalizes blame, you can try to point out that what is shared by all the factors she blames is herself—that she is "the common thread." (Take a look at the sidebar on the facing page to get an idea of how best to communicate this; these guidelines apply here as well as to addressing your mate's attempts to normalize the abnormal.) But don't be surprised if your initial attempt to "connect the dots" is rejected vehemently. And please don't let this discourage you from trying again at another time, possibly even many times.

My husband and I went through this. Seeing what I was doing, he would repeatedly say that the common denominator across all of the situations I blamed for my mood swings was me. For instance, when I would complain about someone at work, he would say, "That's funny, you had the same type of problem with so-and-so last week." When I retorted that a lot of people are difficult to get along with, he said gently, "I know. But do you think it could it be true for everyone you come in contact with—all the people at the university, our neighbors, the guy at the dry cleaning shop, and the cashier at the supermarket?" Although I didn't want to hear it the first (or second or third) time, eventually I did get the message. And this actually was one of the small steps that led to my recognition that I had bipolar disorder.

"It's Not Me; It's You"

Sometimes bipolar people blame the people they are closest to when they are feeling angry, down, or overwhelmed and unable to cope. You may hear, "You made me get like this" or "It's your fault," even though you know you haven't done anything to cause what you're witnessing. Your partner even may project his emotional illness onto you, maintaining that *you* are the one who really has the problem. That's what happened with Ethan and June.

It was Ethan's wife, June, not Ethan, who called to schedule an evaluation for him. On the telephone June relayed how emotionally out of control Ethan had become in recent months, ever since a major business deal of his had gone bad.

On the day of his appointment, when I went to the waiting room to meet him, I found both Ethan and June sitting there. Ethan insisted that June come into the session with him. He walked fast and looked angry as he headed toward my open office door with June and me trailing behind him.

Within a matter of minutes it was clear that Ethan was in a manic episode. He was pacing nonstop around my office, repeatedly and loudly demanding to know whether there were any hidden cameras in the room, getting so upset that while he was talking saliva was actually spewing out of his mouth. But he maintained there was nothing wrong with him. He had agreed to see me along with his wife because, according to Ethan, she had a serious mental health problem. Poor June sat on the couch in my office immobile and silent, looking perplexed and helpless as Ethan raged on about how "mentally ill" she was.

Fortunately, by the end of the session I was able to engage Ethan and form a connection with him. I convinced him to go see a psychiatrist to possibly get some medication that would help him live better in the "stressful circumstances" he was in, that is, in his mind, living with someone with mental health problems. Luckily, the match between the psychiatrist and Ethan was a good one. After only a handful of visits the psychiatrist was able to persuade Ethan to take a mood stabilizer. Today, with Ethan's bipolar disorder under control, he and June are doing well.

In this situation I was able to coax Ethan to get help for himself by building on his way of thinking about things—that he was under stress because of "his wife's mental health problem"—rather than confronting him with the truth. Had I said, "Ethan you're the one with the problem, not June," he probably would have stormed out of my office and wouldn't have ended up getting the help he needed.

If you are in a similar situation, you might try suggesting that the two of you go to see a doctor to address the issues that are on your partner's mind, the ones that are "about you." Once you've gotten your mate in the door, a skilled professional should be able to pick up on what's really going on and, ideally, gently persuade your loved one to get the assistance he or she needs. (I realize this approach may seem somewhat manipulative, but I think its use is warranted in a circumstance like this, where a major mental health problem is going undiagnosed and untreated.)

"It's Not Me; It's Where We're Living"

It is not uncommon for a bipolar person to desire to return to a place or time (or both) before he or she was diagnosed, or when and where he or she was relatively well. (Actually, this desire is not exclusive to people who have bipolar disorder; many with other serious illnesses—psychiatric and other—feel this way too.) People hope that returning to a setting from the past will allow their old selves to reemerge. It's an escape fantasy that's based on denial, or at least minimization, of one's illness.

I went through something like this when I was in a rough period of my illness. I felt that moving back to Pittsburgh, where I had spent the early stages of my career, was the answer to my mood problem. During the Pittsburgh years no one had yet diagnosed me as having bipolar disorder, nor was I on any type of psychiatric medication. I was, as mental health professionals like to say, "high functioning"—productive at work, with a good social life and a great relationship with my husband (I'm glad to be able to say things are this way now too).

So why didn't I move back to Pittsburgh then? Because I knew deep inside that moving back really wouldn't allow me to recapture my former self, that my current self was going to go with me wherever I went. In other words, I couldn't undo the bipolar disorder by changing locations. (Anyway, I had had bipolar disorder back then too, although I didn't—or didn't want to—recognize it at the time.)

Instead of longing to return to a happier time or place, your partner may feel the urge to find a new location, one where everything, it is hoped, will be much better, where the mood problem will go away or become less severe. When people are in the depressed cycles of their bipolar disorder, they are particularly likely to think that moving will make their situation better. (When they're manic, they are more likely to think about changing life partners.) They often consider relocating to exotic destinations (islands, other countries), rural areas here in the United States (to get away from it all), or anyplace that is very far away from where they're currently living (the farther away geographically, the farther away from the disorder).

Of course, since bipolar disorder is at its core a biological illness, an environmental change is not going to cure it. I'm not claiming, though, that one's surroundings can't make a difference. As I discuss in Chapter 7, different aspects of the environment can positively or negatively impact the disorder, as is true of other chronic illnesses too. But while it's possible that there are places that would be a better environmental fit for your partner, unfortunately, there isn't anywhere the two of you can move to get rid of this illness. (And since research shows that moving is one of the five most stressful life events, and stress often precipitates the development of mood episodes, relocating can actually make your partner's illness worse.)

If your partner is pushing for a move, my advice is to say what most mental health professionals advise a patient in crisis: "Don't make a major life decision or change until you're feeling better." This way you're not actually saying no but instead suggesting that the two of you put the idea on hold until your mate is in a better state of mind. When that time comes, you'll be better able to use the methods I described earlier to convince your partner that his mood problem is not caused by outside factors, but rather originating from within.

"That Doctor Doesn't Know What He's Talking About"

As for most psychiatric disorders, a diagnosis of bipolar disorder is based on observation and history, relying heavily on the clinical judgment of the doctor who is performing the diagnostic evaluation. This perceived subjectivity combined with the fact that there are no objective medical tests (like blood tests or X-rays) that can prove your loved one has bipolar disorder can make it easy for your partner to dismiss what the doctor says. That's why, when someone does dismiss the doctor's diagnosis, I often advise **getting at least two (and possibly three) independent diagnostic opinions.** It's easy to reject what one doctor has to say, but much harder to ignore the opinions of multiple doctors who concur.

Remember Marty, described on the first page of this chapter? Marty discounted the bipolar diagnosis his doctor gave him. Let's take a look at how his wife, Sharon, handled the situation.

Marty: That doctor doesn't know what he's talking about. He probably got his degree from some mail-order place!

Sharon: I understand your not wanting to believe you have bipolar disorder based on what this one doctor had to say. I think we should get at least one other opinion—maybe even two more—before we accept that that's what it really is.

Marty: That's a good idea. We'll go see someone else, someone who really knows what he's doing.

Sharon: Right, we'll see a doctor who is tops. We don't want to make a mistake about anything as important as this.

Although Marty's motivation for seeing another doctor really is to disprove or discredit the first doctor's conclusions, Marty will be hard-pressed to continue to deny that he has bipolar disorder if a second doctor comes up with the same diagnosis. It will be even more difficult to deny the second doctor's opinion if Marty has played a role in choosing the second physician. That's why, if you're in a situation like this, I advise you to either have your mate or the two of you together select the doctor who will render the second opinion. And if your partner does deny a second, concurring opinion, suggest a third evaluation—and again make sure your partner is involved in picking the doctor.

In all likelihood your partner will find it hard to argue with the results when the "experiment" produces the same answer two or three times in a row. But if she is still not convinced, try another scientific approach: ***examine whether the disorder runs in your mate's family.*** Since bipolar disorder has a strong genetic component it's possible that one or more of your loved one's relatives has the disorder too. (Of course, this exercise isn't going to be of use if your mate was adopted and has no knowledge of his or her biological relatives. If this is the case, just skip this section of the chapter.) Also, since research has shown that other types of mood disorders, including unipolar depression, have an increased prevalence in the families of people who have bipolar disorder, your partner can expect to find this as well in his family tree.

Show your mate the following questions so that she can think about how they apply to family members. To be thorough, your partner should consider all adult first-degree relatives—mother, father, and full siblings (brothers and sisters), and children too, if they are old enough that this makes sense, as well as second-degree relatives—maternal and paternal grandparents, aunts and uncles, and any half siblings. (Third-degree relatives—like cousins—can also be considered if your partner has enough information about them.)

Your mate can do this exercise alone or together with you if that's comfortable for her. If you and your loved one have been together for a long time, you might even come up with information that your partner has forgotten. Your mate also may want to "fill in the blanks" by obtaining additional information from the relative who is suspected of having a mood problem (if that feels appropriate) or by talking to other family members to see what they know or can recall about that person.

- Are there any relatives who were evaluated or treated by a psychiatrist, psychologist, or other mental health professional? If yes, do you know what the diagnosis was or what they were treated for?
- Were any family members ever hospitalized or "institutionalized" for a psychiatric problem? If yes, do you know what the diagnosis was or why they were there?
- Have any relatives been prescribed psychiatric medication? If yes, do you know what type (antidepressants, tranquilizers, mood stabilizers, etc.) or what for?
- Have any relatives taken their own lives or tried to commit suicide?
- Have any family members had electroconvulsive shock therapy (ECT; often referred to as "shock therapy")?
- Have any relatives had problems with mood swings, depression, or a "nervous breakdown"?
- Have any family members had drug or alcohol problems?

If your mate answers yes to any one of these questions, it is highly likely that that particular relative has a history of some type of psychiatric disorder. The more detailed the information that can be recalled or collected, the better your odds of knowing whether the problem is mood-related or bipolar disorder in particular.

The form below can be used to note which relatives are suspected of having mood disorders and those who may have bipolar disorder. Your partner can either record the findings for all of his or her relatives (in this case you'll probably need an additional copy of the form) or only those who are thought to have a history of a mood disorder. To note the presence of a mood disorder or bipolar disorder your partner can just place a checkmark in the appropriate column.

Although it's very likely that your loved one has at least one relative who has a history of some type of mood disorder, if none can be identified (putting aside the problem of having incomplete information or because there just aren't any clear instances of mood disorder in the family), it could be because another type of psychiatric disorder or other behavior is "masking" the mood disorder. For instance, substance abuse often coexists with mood disorders but makes diagnosing

Mood Disorders in Relatives

Name	Relationship	Mood disorder?	Bipolar disorder?
_____	_____	___	___
_____	_____	___	___
_____	_____	___	___
_____	_____	___	___
_____	_____	___	___
_____	_____	___	___
_____	_____	___	___
_____	_____	___	___

them difficult. Anxiety disorders, like panic and obsessive–compulsive disorders, can conceal the presence of an underlying mood problem.

Your partner needs to know, however, that an absence of mood disorders in biological relatives does not mean that he himself doesn't have bipolar disorder. It just means that there isn't genetic "loading" for the disorder, which may have implications for the treatment and outcome of your partner's illness.

"I'm Just Depressed"

In Chapter 1 I mentioned that bipolar individuals often view their problem as being depression only, not acknowledging their manic or hypomanic periods. So how do you get bipolar people to see that their moods swing in two directions when they hold on to the idea that they have unipolar depression? Having them complete a questionnaire about themselves—specifically about manic/hypomanic symptoms— sometimes helps them accept the truth because it's right there in black and white.

If your partner is agreeable, have her complete the checklist on the facing page. You can do this together with your mate if that's okay with her. It actually can be helpful to your loved one to get your input because her current state of mind, or rather "state of mood," could influence how the questionnaire is filled out. For instance, when people are depressed they may have trouble recalling their manic or hypo- manic times. If this is the situation with your mate, you might tact- fully remind your partner of a period when she was having manic or hypomanic symptoms. For example, "Honey, do you remember that time last summer when you were _____ [really happy, angry all the time, running to the mall every day, etc.]?"

If your partner does not want you to be involved in filling out the checklist, you might just take a look at it to see which items you think apply to your mate but not write down your answers or share them with your partner, because coming up with differing results could lead to unproductive arguments (for example, "What do you mean you think I'm impulsive?!").

I designed this checklist for use in my practice to help people identify and acknowledge the manic and hypomanic symptoms they experience during manic, hypomanic, or mixed episodes. While there is no score that definitively says your mate has had an episode of this

Mood Disorder Checklist

Place a checkmark next to each item that describes or applies to you.

1. ____ Periods when I needed less sleep than usual

2. ____ A history of mood swings

3. ____ Periods of being very "up" or "too happy" for no special reason

4. ____ Periods when I had a lot of intense reactions to situations

5. ____ Periods of being physically agitated—restless, trouble sitting still, or pacing

6. ____ Times of tremendous self-confidence

7. ____ A history of decisions that in retrospect were not sound

8. ____ Periods of great productivity, getting a lot done at school, work, or home

9. ____ Periods when I was excessively irritable or angry and couldn't seem to get along with people

10. ____ Times when my thoughts seemed to be racing through my head

11. ____ Periods when my speech was pressured, like talking too fast or not being able to get the words out fast enough

12. ____ Periods when I found myself acting on impulse a lot

13. ____ Periods when I was easily distracted, couldn't focus on things

14. ____ A history of enjoying taking risks, like excessive gambling, spending sprees that led to a lot of debt, drinking and driving, affairs, dubious investments and business enterprises, etc.

15. ____ Times when I got obsessed with projects, like being a workaholic, staying up till 3:00 A.M. to finish a scrapbook, etc.

16. ____ Periods when I was very outgoing, much more social than usual

17. ____ Periods when I was unusually energetic or more sexual than usual

18. ____ Times when I felt very suspicious or "paranoid"

19. ____ Times when I considered myself a "chosen" person or having a special purpose in life

20. ____ Periods when I was more talkative than usual

From *When Someone You Love Is Bipolar* by Cynthia G. Last. Copyright 2009 by Cynthia G. Last.

type and/or has bipolar disorder (keep in mind that the diagnosis must come from a qualified professional), I can tell you that bipolar individuals generally endorse 10 or more of the items. That doesn't mean, however, that if your mate checks off fewer than 10 that he doesn't have the illness. It just means that he has fewer manic or hypomanic symptoms than some other people who have the disorder. As you'll recall from Chapter 1, only three or four symptoms, in addition to disturbed mood, are needed to qualify as having mania or hypomania (three if the mood is elevated, four if the mood is irritable).

When I met Stewart and his wife, Kyoko, Stewart had already been diagnosed as having bipolar disorder by both a local psychiatrist and a team of mental health professionals at a very well-known psychiatric hospital in another state (one that happens to have a specialty program for bipolar disorder). Unwilling to accept the diagnosis, he came to me to be treated for what he referred to as his "depression." While he certainly had depressive symptoms—crying, loss of interest in all his usual activities, physical agitation, extreme indecisiveness, and thoughts that he'd be better off dead, he had manic ones as well.

Stewart was consumed with the idea that his wife would develop cancer because of X-rays that had been taken prior to a minor surgical procedure. Stewart spoke really fast and forcefully as he recounted all the research he had been doing to discover the link between radiation and cancer. He said he was up till all hours of the night working on this project, getting very little sleep but full of energy for his "mission." As he recounted his story, his mood continuously changed from tearful to joking to angry.

Although it was clear to me, as it had been to the other mental health professionals he had seen, that Stewart was in the midst of a mixed episode of bipolar disorder, he refused to believe he had the disorder because of the presence of his depressive symptoms. Fortunately, having him complete the questionnaire and educating him about mixed episodes—that manic and depressive symptoms can occur at the same time—paid off. He finally was able to see that he did, in fact, have bipolar disorder and ultimately agreed to take the mood-stabilizing medication that had been prescribed for him.

Unfortunately, many doctors do not take the time to talk to their patients about the conditions they have. In some cases it's simply a matter of time—time the doctors don't have. In other instances there's a negative attitude toward giving patients knowledge about their illnesses. (I believe this is a carryover from the way medical care used to be conducted, before people developed the desire to be educated consumers and "took charge" of their own health care.)

The doctor who diagnosed your mate certainly is in a position to educate your loved one about bipolar illness. If the doctor chooses not to do so, or even if the doctor does do so, as I've said throughout this chapter, there's much your mate can do on his own or with your help to learn more about bipolar disorder, acquiring information that can help in accepting the diagnosis.

"Whatever—It's No Big Deal"

Sometimes it's people's attitudes about their diagnoses that show they are minimizing or denying their illness. For example, Tom says, "The doctor is making a bigger deal out of this bipolar thing than it really is." Caitlin thinks, "It's just the mental health profession's way of saying I'm moody."

The problem with attitudes like Tom's and Caitlin's is that making light of the disorder can lead to not getting treatment or being inconsistent with treatment, both of which put people at much greater risk of having additional mood episodes. (Taking medication in a haphazard manner, or stopping it altogether, is a form of denial that people often manifest after they've entered treatment. Not following the doctor's advice about lifestyle changes that are so important to maintaining good mood health is another way individuals minimize their illness.)

"It's no big deal."

"It's mumbo jumbo."

"We all have something wrong with us."

"So what?"

It's not just people who have bipolar disorder who may minimize the diagnosis's importance; family members may do so as well. Just the other day I was talking to a relative of mine about the mood swings another relative has. The first relative, the one without bipolar disorder, said with a huff, "Well, a lot of people are moody—that doesn't mean they have bipolar disorder!"

If your partner already is minimizing or denying the illness, having someone close to her (whose opinion your partner values) voice a similar point of view can make your mate even more resistant to the diagnosis and to getting treatment. So what can you do? You might

consider having a talk with the relative who's downplaying the significance of the illness, letting the individual know that he or she, possibly inadvertently, is strengthening your partner's denial. Part of your
conversation might be aimed at educating the family member (or close
friend) about bipolar illness so that this person can better see that the
kinds of behaviors and emotions your partner experiences fall into this
category.

Another possibility is to consider having the family member
accompany you and your loved one to see the doctor who has diagnosed your partner (this, of course, should be done only with your
loved one's approval, and it is probably appropriate only with the closest relatives, such as a parent or sibling). Hearing the truth about your
mate's illness directly from the doctor may help your partner's relative
accept what the family member hasn't up to that point been able or
willing to face.

What to Do When All Else Fails

I've had very intelligent patients who in the face of overwhelming evidence still have refused to accept that they have bipolar disorder. And,
unfortunately, some of them are still suffering today, much more than
they need to, because of their inability to accept the truth.

As I've said before in this book (and as I'll continue to say in future
chapters when it's relevant), no one wants to have bipolar disorder. I
know I certainly didn't, and, as I also said earlier, it took me several
years after I was first diagnosed to believe it was true. If this can happen to a psychologist who diagnoses and treats bipolar illness, I think
it could, unfortunately, happen to your partner as well.

What do you do if you've tried everything I've outlined in the
preceding pages and you're still where you began—with a partner who
just plain refuses to accept that it's bipolar disorder? This is what happened to my patient Arnold.

Arnold admits that he has mood swings, but he does not, according to him, have bipolar disorder. Yes, he agrees, his mother had
manic–depression, as does his brother. And now his son Max has been
diagnosed with the illness as well.

I have treated Arnold on and off for many years, and although
there's no question he's doing much, much better than when I first

met him (at which time he was contemplating suicide), to this day he denies that he has the disorder that runs in his family. The weight of the genetic evidence plus his own symptoms didn't lead him to the obvious conclusion because it was too painful for him to accept that he was like the other members of his family. And although I was able to help him with therapy, and to work with his wife on ways she could help him too, he undoubtedly could have gotten more relief from his illness if he had accepted the diagnosis and gotten medication for it.

Arnold is an example of someone who, no matter what tack the people around him take, may never admit to having bipolar disorder. On the other hand, he might simply need more time to accept his situation. If I could accept the truth after years of denial, then Arnold might be able to too. But if he doesn't, there are still many things his loved ones can do to help him, just as you can help your mate, and the two of you as a couple, to have a better life right now. It all starts with getting the right treatment, the subject of the next chapter.

4

What You Need to Know about Your Partner's Treatment

Tamara's "nervous breakdown" was the scariest experience of her life. Thank goodness her husband, David, and their family doctor were able to talk her into seeing a psychiatrist, who, after spending several sessions with her, diagnosed Tamara with bipolar disorder. Although it wasn't always easy, during the next 6 months Tamara was diligent while the doctor tried her on several different combinations of medication, eventually getting her treatment regimen just right.

Although Tamara is grateful she's so much better now, the drugs have side effects that are really hard to deal with. She's started speculating about whether she could take fewer medications or lower doses, or possibly even stop taking them altogether and go for therapy instead.

David doesn't know how to respond to his wife's concern. Does she really need to be on so many different medications? Are the side effects something she just has to get used to? Aren't there other treatment options, and, if so, why hasn't the doctor tried them?

David's wife has a serious medical illness, and he knows very little about how it is treated. That's understandable: bipolar disorder isn't particularly common. But he could relieve a lot of his own stress and improve his life, his wife's life, and their life together as a couple by reading up on the illness to learn some specifics about the different treatment options that are available to Tamara.

Reading this chapter, David would discover that people with bipolar disorder frequently require multiple medications and that the drugs need to be taken on a regular basis even in the absence of active symptoms. He would learn that medication side effects often go away with time and that when they don't physicians are likely to prescribe reductions in drug dosages or change the medications. He'd find out that therapy can be very useful in helping to manage the illness but that it is an adjunct to medical treatment, not a substitute. Finally, he would know about the whole range of treatments we are now fortunate to have available for this disorder. (And if he continued reading in the future, he'd learn about new treatments as they become available too.)

Although for centuries people with bipolar disorder had to suffer without hope of relief, today we are in a very exciting time, a time when there are a great many effective treatment options. And with these options come choices, choices you, your partner, and your partner's doctor can make together. That's why it's so important that you—like David—learn about these different treatments—how and for whom they work, what their benefits are, and what disadvantages or side effects may come into play. With this knowledge you can help guide and support your mate through some critical decisions, those that will have a major impact on your partner's life and your life together.

Because psychiatric medications play such a major role in bipolar health, you and your partner are going to want to make sure you not only know something about these drugs but also find the right physician to manage the medical aspect of your loved one's care. That's why I begin this chapter by discussing how you can go about locating a professional who will not only have the expertise necessary to treat your mate, but the compassion and other characteristics that are so valuable as well.

Finding the Right Doctor

If your loved one already has been diagnosed by a physician (or other professional who has prescribing privileges) whom he or she is comfortable with, your mate may want to continue with that doctor for treatment. But if the initial diagnosis was given by a psychologist or your partner isn't sure the current doctor is the right one for him or her, you'll want to seek out a doctor who not only has the necessary medical expertise but also has the other traits that make for a good doctor–patient fit.

I offer the following suggestions *to you* because in my experience many people with bipolar disorder benefit from, or require, the help of their partners in finding a doctor. People who are actively manic or hypomanic, for example, often are not motivated to seek the help they clearly need. But they might agree to see a doctor if someone else finds the doctor, makes the appointment, and possibly agrees to go along. On the other hand, those who are severely depressed may desperately desire help but be incapable of doing the research or getting a referral, calling the doctor's office, driving to the appointment, and so forth. And even if your loved one is willing and able to handle this task, he still may value your input.

Incidentally, when I use the term *doctor* in this section, I'm referring to a physician or medical doctor, either an MD or a DO—those professionals who can prescribe medicine, not a PhD (which is the degree that many psychologists, including me, have).

Psychiatrists and Psychopharmacologists

Psychiatrists are physicians (medical doctors, or MDs) who have specialized after medical school, during residency, in psychiatry. When they complete their residency training, most take a series of tests that, if passed, qualifies them as "board certified in psychiatry and neurology" (neurology is an integral part of the psychiatry residency but not its primary focus, as would be the case for neurologists). Board certification means that a certain standard of clinical competency has been obtained, and, because of this, I strongly suggest that when you look for a psychiatrist (or psychopharmacologist for that matter) you select one who has met this criterion.

Psychiatrists prescribe medication, but some of them also offer therapy services as part of their medication visits or even do therapy by itself. Although I know it's a generalization, it's been my experience, both personally and professionally, that psychiatrists who do therapy in addition to or as part of managing medication tend to be warmer and seem more caring. They also tend to spend more time with their patients, typically 20 to 30 minutes for a medication visit, as opposed to the alternative 10-minute "in and out the door" visit that doesn't really allow adequate time for questions or discussion of current concerns.

Most psychiatrists treat bipolar disorder. Those who focus their work in this area often are affiliated with university- or hospital-based specialty programs, but there are many private practitioners who have extensive experience with the illness too who are equipped to treat bipolar individuals. You can start your search in several different ways—via word of mouth from people you know, a referral from your family doctor, or research conducted on the Web (many doctors have their own websites, or they have spots on the websites of hospitals or universities they are affiliated with). You also can visit bipolar websites (see Resources), some of which have lists of doctors who specialize in treating bipolar disorder.

Sandy and Charles spent a lot of time looking for just the right doctor to treat Charles's bipolar disorder. They wanted a psychiatrist who not only had a lot of experience with the illness but also would take the time to talk to Charles about how he was doing, not just write a prescription and quickly send him on his way.

When they found Dr. Scott (not the doctor's real name), they knew he was exactly what they had been searching for. Not only does he specialize in bipolar disorder; the doctor is warm and compassionate and spends more time with Charles than any of the other psychiatrists he's seen before. When Sandy accompanies Charles to an appointment, Dr. Scott always welcomes her to join them and answers all of her questions. And if they need to get in touch with him after hours, he calls them back right away.

Charles had to go through several doctors, as your mate might too, before he found the one who was right for him, one that met the following criteria:

- Experienced in treating bipolar disorder
- Caring and empathetic
- Spends adequate time during visits
- Open to questions
- Comfortable with having spouse/partner involved in treatment
- Can be reached in an emergency

Finding the Right Doctor: What to Look For

- Ask people you trust for the name of a good psychiatrist or psychopharmacologist—such as friends who have been pleased with their own choice of doctor or your internist or family doctor. If you can't obtain a referral, find your own by surfing the Internet (see Resources for sites that can help with this).

- If the doctor has a website, or is affiliated with a hospital or university and included on its website, or you can get a copy of the doctor's CV, examine the *credentials* that are listed:
  - Did the doctor go to a well-known and respected medical school?
  - How about the residency program?
  - Is the doctor board certified in psychiatry?
  - Did the doctor do a fellowship after completing his or her residency? If yes, what did it specialize in?
  - Is the doctor a member (in good standing) of the American Psychiatric Association? Does the doctor belong to any other national or regional professional organizations?

- Does the doctor have *staff privileges* at at least one local hospital?

- Does the doctor have any *clinical or academic appointments,* like clinical or adjunct faculty at a university or head of a department of psychiatry at a local hospital or mental health facility?

- Before scheduling an appointment, try to *speak at least briefly with the doctor* on the telephone (if this isn't possible, speak with the office manager):
  - Does the doctor have a mostly adult practice?
  - What percentage consists of bipolar individuals? Does the doctor have a particular interest in bipolar disorder?
  - Does the doctor do therapy in addition to prescribing medication?
  - How long is the initial visit, and how long are follow-up visits?
  - What is the doctor's availability after hours and on weekends?

Like Charles, I think all of the preceding are important in selecting a psychiatrist. It's possible, though, that your partner isn't interested in "hand-holding" or spending more time than necessary for medication checks. Your mate may want an expert and not really care about the personality that comes along with that individual's expertise. People who feel this way may turn to psychopharmacologists for their medication.

Like psychiatrists, psychopharmacologists are medical doctors (MDs) who have specialized in psychiatry. Since the residency programs are the same—a specialization in psychiatry—for both psychiatrists and psychopharmacologists, it really is important to know what extra training any doctor may have had that qualifies him or her to use this title. Since there is no certification process or licensing requirement for claiming that one is a psychopharmacologist, you or your partner (or the two of you) need to look at the doctor's background and credentials to determine the extent of his or her expertise. (One way to do this is to ask for a copy of the doctor's *curriculum vitae*, or CV, the term used to describe what is referred to as a *résumé* in other circles.)

Physicians who put themselves forth as being psychopharmacologists almost always deal exclusively with medication—they do not do therapy. Because they don't do therapy, visits tend to be brief, often 10 to 15 minutes (but as I mentioned before, there are psychiatrists too who do their "medication checks" in this amount of time), except for the initial evaluation, which can span from 45 to 90 minutes.

A good psychopharmacologist may be, and I stress *may be*, more creative and innovative in approaching your loved one's pharmacological treatment. Psychopharmacologists often are known for thinking "outside the box" and coming up with unique "medication cocktails." However, as I said earlier, since there's no set standard for people using this title, you and your mate will have to rely on a referral from someone you trust and/or do the homework on your own.

Family Doctors

Some people with bipolar disorder prefer to be treated by their family doctors. Is your partner uncomfortable with the stigma she perceives is associated with seeing a "shrink"? Perhaps she wishes to downplay the significance of her illness ("It's not that bad that I need a psy-chiatrist") or just feels more comfortable sharing private information about her mental health with someone she's known for some time.

Although it's common practice today for physicians who don't spe-cialize in psychiatry to prescribe psychiatric medications, in the case of bipolar disorder this may not be the best way to go, particularly if your partner has not yet been diagnosed. Family doctors may be able to pick up on depression, but because they haven't studied psychiatry (other than a course or two in medical school), they may lack the expertise needed to formulate a bipolar disorder diagnosis. And without the cor-rect diagnosis, your partner won't receive the right treatment.

If your loved one hasn't yet been diagnosed and does go see his family physician during the depressed phase of his illness, it's likely that the doctor will give a diagnosis of depression and then prescribe an antidepressant. The problem with this is that virtually all antide-pressants risk "overshooting the mark" in a person who has bipolar tendencies, causing the development of manic, mixed, or hypomanic episodes, also known as "the manic switch." (That's why, as I discuss later in this chapter, antidepressants used to treat bipolar disorder typ-ically are given in combination with a mood-stabilizing drug.)

This is what happened to 29-year-old Gail. Although she had battled ups and downs throughout her 20s, she had never tried medi-cation for her mood disorder, fearful that the drugs would "mess with her mind." But now in a very severe depressed episode, she was finally open to the idea of giving medication a try. Uncomfortable with the idea of seeing a psychiatrist, she went to her internist instead.

Gail left her internist's office with a prescription for an antide-pressant and after 2 weeks on the medication was hypomanic. At the time she didn't know she was hypomanic; she just knew she was feel-ing really, really great and figured this is how people who don't suffer from depression probably feel most of the time.

Since her hypomania wasn't that impairing, the "high" Gail got from the antidepressant wasn't as terrible as it might have been for someone whose functioning or judgment gets significantly affected by an elevated state. But what was awful for Gail was that after a couple of months of being "up" she landed back where she started—depressed but now with some loss of hope, the hope she had had for a pharmacological cure. (Just to let you know, several months later Gail was willing to give medication a try again. This time, though, she went to a psychiatrist and got the medication that was right for her condition.)

Despite the reservations I've shared with you, I have to say that if the only way you can get your mate into the health care system is by seeing the family doctor, by all means do so. At least your partner is admitting there's a problem and is willing to get help. This is a first step that, it is hoped, will eventually lead your mate to move on, with the encouragement of the family doctor, to a physician who specializes in psychiatry.

It is, however, very important for people to visit their family physicians *before* beginning treatment (even if this doctor isn't the one who is going to be administering the psychiatric medication) to rule out an organic, as opposed to a psychiatric, cause for the mood swings (see Chapter 2). It's also an opportunity to get baseline (pretreatment) measures on different aspects of overall physical health so that any changes that occur as a result of treatment can be monitored.

What You Need to Know about Your Partner's Medication

Although the most effective treatment approach for bipolar disorder has several components, medication is undoubtedly the single most important. This is not to minimize the contributions that psychotherapy and self-help strategies can make to wellness. But without medication the benefits your loved one can glean from these are lessened considerably.

Despite the professional advice I obtained, and my own knowledge about bipolar illness, I didn't accept this fact easily. Actually, although it was my own idea to seek out medical treatment for my mood disorder, I ended up having a tremendous problem with the idea that I *had to* be on medication. I took it as a sign of personal failure that I needed to take drugs to be like other people—people who don't have mood swings.

Because the concept of being on medication on a regular basis was so difficult for me, I tried to talk my psychiatrist into treating me for individual mood episodes as they occurred rather than being on maintenance medication (medication all the time). Contrary to her advice, during the early years of my treatment I would from time to time go off my medication, only to find that I ended up in a mood episode once again. Finally, after this had happened one time too many, I recognized that even though I *could* go for periods of time without medication the final result *wasn't* worth it. Really, it was silly, in a way, to try to "prove" that I could manage without something my brain obviously needed to function optimally. I wouldn't try to persuade a diabetic person to prove he could go without insulin, nor would I try to persuade someone on blood pressure medicine to show she could manage without her drug. Why, then, would I risk my health and well-being in a way I wouldn't expect of others?

Like me, your partner may struggle with the idea of not being in "perfect" (mental) health and having to take medication to be well. But perhaps your loved one can take some comfort from knowing that this illness is largely hereditary—that it was nothing she did that caused her to have bipolar disorder. Unlike other serious illnesses that can be linked to unhealthy lifestyle choices (for example, smoking and lung cancer), your mate is not responsible for having this particular illness. What you also need to make sure to convey, though, is that even if there's nothing your partner can do about having been predisposed to this illness, there's plenty she can do to stay as well as possible now that she has it. And staying well means, among other things, taking medication exactly as prescribed each and every day of her life.

While it is beyond the scope of this book to provide an exhaustive account of every psychiatric medication used with bipolar individuals, this chapter gives you an overview of the main classes of medications, as well as more detailed information on some of the specific drugs that are used more frequently, so you will have a greater understanding of the medical aspect of your partner's treatment. For more information on any particular drug, your partner's doctor is a good resource. Also, many of the pharmaceutical companies have websites for the medications they manufacture that may address questions you two have.

One aspect of the medications that I spend a fair amount of time on is side effects. As you'll learn in Chapter 6, bothersome side effects are one of the main reasons that many people discontinue their bipolar medications. I think it's important for you to be aware of any changes and challenges that your partner might experience as part of treatment, because your observations and insight can help encourage your mate to stick with the medication (when that's appropriate) that improves life for both of you.

I talk about the medications or classes of medications one by one because it's easier to organize the material that way, but please don't assume this means that when I describe a medication's benefits I mean to suggest that this, or any, single drug should "do it all" for your partner. Most people with bipolar disorder take multiple medications (like Tamara, introduced at the beginning of this chapter) to keep their illness in check. It's not unusual for someone to be on three, four, five, or even more drugs at the same time, and the number of medications doesn't necessarily reflect the severity of your loved one's illness. It's also probably a good idea to read the whole section on medications even if you don't recognize many of the drug names as part of your partner's current treatment regimen, to familiarize yourself with all the different treatment options available.

Although some people find the medications that are effective for them early on, soon after starting treatment, others—like Tamara— have to go through multiple medication trials before finding the right drug or combination of drugs. This can be a very difficult process for both of you. Tamara's husband, David, tried to be upbeat and positive around his wife through each and every medication trial. But inwardly he really was anxious and worried, fearful that Tamara would have another "nervous breakdown" before getting a chance to recover completely from the first one. Fortunately, David's fear wasn't realized. Although it took 6 months for Tamara and her doctor to arrive at the right combination of drugs, she "held it together" for the entire period and eventually felt like her old self again.

Although huge strides have been made in psychopharmacology, the science simply isn't yet at the point where doctors can know with certainty which medicines your partner will respond to. Therefore, a certain amount of trial and error is almost inevitable. Medication guidelines known as *decision trees* or *algorithms* established by various professional organizations (like the American Psychiatric Association) help steer doctors in the right direction, and to these guidelines physicians add their wealth of clinical experience to arrive at the best prescription decisions. Nevertheless, I think most experts would agree that psychopharmacology is still in its infancy when compared to other areas of medicine.

Someday, I hope, doctors will be able to perform a simple blood test to determine which brain chemicals a person has too much or too little of and then prescribe a medication to restore the proper balance.

But until that time anyone with bipolar disorder may suffer disappointments on the road to recovery. In Chapter 6 I'll talk at length about getting over these stumbling blocks. For now, please try to stay hopeful, keeping in mind that your mate should, like countless others, eventually achieve mood stability by sticking with the medication trials.

Mood Stabilizers

For decades mood stabilizers have been the mainstay of pharmacological treatment for bipolar disorder. Mood stabilizers do exactly what the term implies: they keep bipolar moods from getting too high or too low. They are used both in the treatment of acute mood episodes (episodes that already are under way) and as a maintenance medication (as a preventative).

Lithium

Of all the medications currently used to treat bipolar illness, **lithium** has the longest history. As a result we have a lot of research data on its efficacy. Decades of studies clearly show that lithium is not only effective in the treatment of acute mania and, to a slightly lesser degree, acute bipolar depression but also has a prophylactic effect—it reduces the frequency, duration, and severity of future episodes of mania and depression and dramatically reduces the risk of suicide (which, as noted in Chapter 2, is disproportionately high among bipolar individuals). Lithium carbonate—for example, **Eskalith, Lithobid**—is the most commonly prescribed form of lithium, so when I say *lithium* this is the medication I mean.

Although lithium is a "miracle drug" for many, not everyone with bipolar disorder is a "lithium responder." People who have mixed episodes of illness and/or have the rapid-cycling form of bipolar disorder may not benefit from the drug. On the other hand, if your partner has the "classic" or pure form of mania—including a euphoric mood and grandiose behavior—a positive response to lithium is more likely.

Lithium can take anywhere from 10 days to 3 weeks to work. Doctors will determine whether your partner's dose of lithium is in the "therapeutic range" by measuring the level of the substance in the bloodstream, because people taking the same dose of lithium can have different blood levels. Early in treatment these blood tests are performed frequently to ensure that the level is at a point where it will be effective and, most important, *not too high*, since lithium at high doses can be toxic. The blood lithium level usually is kept between 0.8 and 1.0 millimoles (mmol)/liter, although some research suggests that levels between 0.6 and 0.8 (or even lower) may be effective for maintenance treatment. Finding the lowest effective blood level is important not only to avoid toxicity but because side effects are very much related to blood level. Lithium toxicity usually is associated with blood levels higher than 1.5 mmol/liter. (Many drugs—including, to name just two, nonsteroidal anti-inflammatory drugs and diuretics—increase lithium levels and, consequently, increase the likelihood of toxicity. Your partner's doctor should provide your loved one with a list of medications that interact with lithium in this way.) You need to know, though, that it's possible to experience the effects of toxicity even at a therapeutic blood level, so it's important to know the warning signs of lithium intoxication (see the sidebar below). *If lithium toxicity is suspected, your partner must go to the emergency room to get the proper treatment for this condition.*

Lithium Toxicity: Know the Warning Signs

Gastrointestinal symptoms:	Severe nausea or vomiting
	Diarrhea or incontinence
Muscle coordination problems:	Severe tremor
	Muscle weakness
	Unstable walk
	Muscle twitches
	Slurred speech
	Visual changes (blurred vision; nystagmus)
Altered consciousness:	Inability to concentrate
	Sleepiness
	Confusion or disorientation
	Seizure
	Coma

After the correct dose of medicine has been established, your partner will usually have his lithium blood level checked every 3 to 6 months. Tests of kidney and thyroid functioning also may be performed at these times. Although damage to the kidneys is rare—it tends to occur with toxicity or very high blood levels of the drug for extended periods of time—many physicians still will monitor this to be on the safe side. A reduction in thyroid functioning (hypothyroidism) is more common (estimates range from 5 to 35%) and, when it occurs, is treated with thyroid hormone medications.

As mentioned above, the lower the blood level, the less likely or less severe the side effects of lithium. Some of the drug's side effects tend to be common and difficult for people to tolerate. It's not unusual for people on lithium to complain of a "mental sluggishness" (in psychiatry this is referred to as cognitive dulling)—that they're not as sharp as they used to be. Also, as mentioned in Chapter 2, artistic individuals sometimes report being less creative on the drug. For example, Ian, who used to write music lyrics as a hobby before getting ill, says he can't do this on lithium. However, since he's had "black manias" (psychotic manic episodes that are extremely terrifying, not at all euphoric), he's willing to accept the trade-off.

Decreased coordination is another side effect that's frequently reported. People report feeling clumsier or less agile than they used to be. Weight gain, fine tremor of the hands (which may be treated by using beta-blocker medication), nausea, diarrhea, increased thirst and urination, and exacerbations of preexisting dermatological conditions also occur not uncommonly.

Anticonvulsants

Although anticonvulsant medications weren't initially developed for bipolar disorder—they were first approved for use in treating epilepsy—many of them were discovered to have mood-stabilizing effects. The exact manner by which these drugs affect mood (and epilepsy for that matter) is unknown, but it's speculated that their therapeutic action may have to do with inhibiting excitatory neurotransmitters in the brain.

Depakote is commonly prescribed by psychiatrists for the treatment of acute mania and depression and also as a maintenance therapy. Research suggests it may be particularly beneficial if your loved

What You Need to Know about Mood Stabilizers

- Used for both the acute and maintenance treatment of mania and depression.
- For many of these drugs, therapeutic "dose" is determined by blood levels, so blood tests are necessary.
- Often used in combination with one another to obtain complete symptom remission.
- Side effects can be difficult to tolerate.

one has mixed mood episodes or rapid cycling or has not responded to lithium. The drug also is often used in combination with lithium in people who have not responded completely to lithium alone. Gavin is one of these people.

Gavin's problems began when he started graduate school. In a strange city with unfamiliar people and a very heavy course curriculum, Gavin was under tremendous stress. But the way he behaved went well beyond any typical reaction to stress. He was sending his girlfriend, Sheila, strange e-mails that didn't make sense and calling her at all hours of the night. Worried about him, Sheila traveled to Gavin's university, where she found that, besides not sleeping, he was not eating or showering and didn't want to leave his apartment.

Fortunately, Gavin did not resist when Sheila insisted they see the psychiatrist at the university health center. The doctor started Gavin on lithium, and after a few weeks he was somewhat better—taking better care of himself and willing to leave his home—but the insomnia and racing, "jumbled up" thoughts continued to plague him. The psychiatrist then added Depakote to Gavin's medication regimen. Though it took some time to find the optimal dose (blood levels) of both medications, eventually, in time, Gavin responded completely and was able to return to his graduate work.

Depakote has some advantages over lithium. In the treatment of acute manic episodes it works faster, in days rather than weeks. The drug also has fewer side effects and is less likely to cause toxicity. Among the potential side effects, as with lithium, weight gain is relatively common. Some people experience stomach upset, sleepiness, or mild tremor of the hands; hair loss also can occur. As in treatment with lithium, regular blood tests are performed to measure blood levels of the drug; at these times tests also may be conducted to assess liver functioning (liver inflammation is a very rare side effect), as well as levels of ammonia and certain pancreaic enzymes that can elevate as a result of treatment.

In recent years, the anticonvulsant **Lamictal** has gotten a lot of attention for its effectiveness in treating bipolar depression. In fact, research indicates that Lamictal's antidepressant action is superior to that of lithium and Depakote, and as compared to traditional antidepressants it's much less likely to cause a mood switch into mania.

Lamictal generally has fewer and milder side effects than many of the other mood stabilizers, and when they occur they often go away in time. The most common side effects include headache, dizziness, and sleepiness. Unlike lithium and Depakote, Lamictal doesn't require regular blood level monitoring.

However, there is one potential problem with this drug that you

Mood Stabilizers

Brand name	Pharmaceutical name
Eskalith, Lithobid, Lithonate, Lithotabs	lithium carbonate
Anticonvulsants	
Depakote, Depakene	divalproex sodium, valproate, valproic acid
Dilantin	phenytoin
Gabitril	tiagabine
Keppra	levetiracetam
Lamictal	lamotrigine
Mysoline	primidone
Neurontin	gabapentin
Tegretol	carbamazepine
Topamax	topiramate
Trileptal	oxcarbazepine
Zonegran	zonisamide

and your mate should be aware of—the possibility of developing a dangerous rash. *If your partner develops any kind of rash while taking this medication, immediately contact the doctor.* The risk of this rash can be greatly reduced, though, by the physician's very gradually increasing the dose of the drug over a number of weeks.

Atypical Antipsychotics

A relatively new class of drugs first emerged in 1990 and has since played a major role in the treatment of bipolar disorder. These medications are referred to as "atypical" or "second-generation" because they are newer than and act somewhat differently from the "typical" or "first-generation" antipsychotics discussed in the following section. They are much more widely used than their predecessors for a couple of reasons:

1. They are as effective as the traditional antipsychotics in treating psychotic symptoms (delusions and hallucinations) and the agitation or hyperactivity that accompanies severe mood episodes but, because they're less strong inhibitors of dopamine, they are thought to carry less of a risk of a particular movement-related side effect ("tardive dyskinesia") that the typical antipsychotics do.
2. They are effective for treating acute episodes of mania and depression, have been shown to prevent future mood episodes (which is why, as you can see from the sidebar on page 110, both **Zyprexa** and **Abilify**—two of the drugs in this class—have been approved by the Food and Drug Administration [FDA] as maintenance treatments for bipolar disorder), and work for mixed episodes and rapid-cycling forms of bipolar disorder.

For these reasons, atypical antipsychotics are evolving into the new standard for long-term treatment of bipolar disorder, *even in individuals with no history of psychosis.* So please understand that taking one of these "antipsychotic" drugs does not necessarily mean your mate is psychotic.

Another advantage of the atypical antipsychotics over the traditional mood stabilizers (with the exception of **Clozaril**) is that blood tests are not needed to adjust dosage or monitor for potential toxicity or other medical consequences. They also are not as likely to cause interactions with other drugs.

Some of the atypical antipsychotics—Clozaril, **Seroquel,** and Zyprexa—are, however, very sedating. These three drugs also are known for their tendency to put weight on people and to cause "metabolic syndrome" (see Chapter 2), with Zyprexa being the worst in this regard (it's worth pointing out, though, that weight gain on Zyprexa may be dose related—the lower the dose, the less weight people generally gain). Research indicates that Abilify and **Geodon,** on the other hand, may not cause these side effects and possibly are as effective as mood stabilizers.

Fifty-five years old and having had bipolar disorder virtually all of her adult life, over the years Margaret had seen many psychiatrists and been tried on almost all of the traditional mood stabilizers without success. Although she was pessimistic about meeting yet another doctor and perhaps being disappointed once again, she eventually agreed to see one of the psychiatrists I refer to. The physician prescribed Zyprexa, and after just 2 short weeks her response was nothing short of miraculous. Her rapid-cycling mood swings—from rage-filled manias to hopeless, despairing depressions—virtually vanished.

But as her months of treatment on the drug increased, so did her weight. She went from a size 8 to a size 14 in less than 6 months. Unable to tolerate this, she pleaded with her doctor to try her on another medication that might work just as well. Although we all—her psychiatrist, her husband, and I—were concerned about her switching medications, Margaret was relentless in her quest for an alternative. Eventually she was tried on two other atypical antipsychotics, both of which failed to work for her.

Suffering terribly, she finally agreed to go back on Zyprexa and, as everyone hoped, she responded extremely well once more. This time, though, Margaret took on the weight issue full force by committing to an exercise program and reducing her intake of sweets. Not only did she stop putting on the pounds, but she actually lost 15!

There are several points that I hope you will take from this story (and please don't misinterpret me as saying that all bipolar people should be on Zyprexa—even if I were in a position to make a medical recommendation, which I'm not, I wouldn't suggest this). One is that there is a great deal of specificity regarding responses to psychiatric drugs. That is, even drugs from the same class, although

---

What You Need to Know
about Atypical Antipsychotics

- To a large extent, they have replaced typical antipsychotics in the treatment of psychosis.
- Also used in acute and maintenance treatment of bipolar disorder for their mood-stabilizing properties.
- Work for mixed episodes and rapid cyclers.
- Side effects vary by specific drug—the more sedating ones are known to cause weight gain and metabolic syndrome.
- For most, blood tests aren't necessary.

---

similar in their structure and function, are not identical and will not necessarily work equally well for a particular individual. (That's why it's not unusual for people to have to try out several medications *even in the same drug class* before arriving at one that works well for them.)

Another point, one that reflects an especially tough situation for the significant others of bipolar individuals, is that your partner may not view the cost–benefit ratio for the medication in the same way you do and, as a result, may want to switch drugs even though it's apparent to you (and the doctors) that this is not in your loved one's best interest. In my experience, when people with this disorder are doing well, they have a short memory for previous mood episodes, so they may not appreciate how far they've come and realize the potential risks associated with making medication changes.

Although switching medications wasn't the solution for Margaret, it frequently is the answer for others. When Howard changed from Seroquel to Geodon, he lost the 20 pounds he had gained from the first drug and his mood continued to stay level. However, since Geodon is not as sedating as Seroquel (in fact, Seroquel is so sedating that it's often used for insomnia that does not respond to traditional prescription sleep medications), his doctor then had to add a tranquilizer (see the section in this chapter on benzodiazepines) to his medication regimen to treat his anxiety symptoms.

Atypical Antipsychotics

Brand name	Pharmaceutical name
Abilify	aripiprazole
Clozaril	clozapine
Geodon	ziprasidone
Risperdal	risperidone
Seroquel	quetiapine
Zeldox	ziprasidone
Zyprexa	olanzapine

Typical Antipsychotics

Typical antipsychotics may be used on a short-term, emergency basis to treat psychosis and extreme hyperactivity or agitation during a severe bipolar episode. In addition to having an antipsychotic effect, these drugs have an almost immediate sedating effect (for this reason, they are sometimes referred to as "major tranquilizers"). The medications can be administered intramuscularly, with an injection, to work even more rapidly.

All medications in this class work by blocking the neurotransmitter dopamine, and the side effects (referred to as *anticholinergic*) commonly experienced are related to this—dry mouth, constipation, and blurred vision. Of greater concern are the variety of movement-related

---

What You Need to Know
about the Typical Antipsychotics

- Used to treat psychotic symptoms and/or extreme hyperactivity or agitation during acute, severe mania or depression.
- Calming effects of the medications work virtually immediately.
- Generally used only short term for bipolar individuals.
- Risk of serious side effects, especially from long-term use.

Typical Antipsychotics

Brand name	Pharmaceutical name
Haldol	haloperidol
Loxitane	loxapine
Mellaril	thioridazine
Moban	molindone
Navane	thiothixene
Prolixin	fluphenazine
Serentil	mesoridazine
Stelazine	trifluoperazine
Thorazine	chlorpromazine
Trilafon	perphenazine

problems (called *extrapyramidal* side effects; see the sidebar below) that can occur, the most worrisome of which is tardive dyskinesia, a condition involving repetitive involuntary movements usually of the facial muscles. While the other movement-related side effects usually can be managed by reducing the dose of medication or administering an anti-Parkinson medication, the only way to get rid of tardive dys-

Movement-Related **Side Effects** of Typical Antipsychotics

"Pseudoparkinsonism":	Slow, shuffling walk; loss of facial expression; trembling of the hands
Dystonic reactions:	Muscle spasms of the face or neck or facialocular muscles
Akathisia:	Intense restlessness in the legs that triggers the need to walk or pace
Tardive dyskinesia:	Repetitive involuntary movements usually of the facial muscles—chewing, blinking, lip pursing, tongue thrusting

kinesia is to stop the medication. (In some cases, even after stopping the medication, tardive dyskinesia can persist and be irreversible.) For this reason, typical antipsychotics have largely been replaced by the atypicals, which studies show are as effective but, as I said earlier, may not carry the same risk of severe movement-related side effects (or anticholinergic ones either).

In practice, however, typical antipsychotics continue to be used by some physicians because they believe, on the basis of clinical experience, that they are the best treatment choice for extreme manic excitability in the most severely disturbed patients. Another consideration that some clinicians take into account is how inexpensive typical antipsychotics are relative to their newer counterparts.

Antidepressants

Antidepressants are used to treat acute episodes of bipolar depression and to prevent new episodes from developing. The use of these drugs for bipolar disorder is somewhat controversial for two reasons:

1. All antidepressants (although they vary in their comparable risks of this) can instigate a manic switch in people with bipolar tendencies.
2. Research indicates that antidepressants increase mood cycling—that is, they decrease the time between mood episodes.

Despite these potential problems, antidepressants remain widely prescribed for bipolar depression. Psychiatrists generally deal with the mood instability aspects of these drugs by using those that are known to have a lower manic switch rate—like **Wellbutrin** or **Paxil**—and/or administering the drug in conjunction with a mood-stabilizing drug (a traditional mood stabilizer or an atypical antipsychotic with mood-stabilizing properties). In fact, most experts in this field agree that *antidepressants should not be administered to people with bipolar disorder in the absence of a mood-stabilizing drug.*

The different types of antidepressants and the specific drugs included in each category are listed in the table on page 109. I've tried to be very inclusive here, but you should know that some of these medications are not used very commonly today, at least in the treatment of bipolar disorder. For example, the **tricyclic antidepressants,** although they have a longer history of use than any of the other antidepressants, are used infrequently today because there now are other equally effective antidepressants available that have fewer side effects and also are less likely to precipitate a manic switch. The **monoamine oxidase inhibitor (MAOI) antidepressants** also are not used widely, primarily because they require certain dietary restrictions. This is unfortunate since research suggests they may be quite effective for a subset of depressed bipolar people—particularly those with bipolar II depressions that have an atypical pattern of symptoms (lack of energy, slowed motor behavior, increased sleep and appetite) and have not responded to other antidepressant drugs. However, there is a relatively new delivery system for this drug—the transdermal (skin) patch—that at low doses does not require people to follow a special diet, so we now are beginning to see an increase in the use of this medication.

Perhaps the most widely known antidepressants are the *SSRIs,* which target primarily the neurotransmitter serotonin (a brain chemical that's related to feelings of well-being) and include such drugs as **Prozac, Zoloft,** Paxil, and **Lexapro.** Also prescribed very commonly is Wellbutrin, an atypical antidepressant that works on the brain chemicals norepinephrine and dopamine and tends to be more energizing in its antidepressant effect (and less likely to cause sexual side effects or weight gain) than the SSRIs. The *SSNRIs,* which affect both serotonin and norepinephrine, have also gained popularity. The medications in these three classes generally have few or mild side effects (see the sidebar on page 108) and also do not require blood tests to establish dose or monitor for adverse medical consequences.

What You Need to Know about Antidepressants

- Used to treat acute episodes of bipolar depression and as a maintenance therapy to prevent new episodes from forming.
- Should be administered in conjunction with a mood- stabilizing drug.
- The newer antidepressants generally are well tolerated.
- For most, blood tests not required.

Common **Side Effects** of Antidepressants

Change in sexual functioning (decreased libido or difficulty obtaining an orgasm)

Weight gain

Insomnia

Daytime sedation

Nausea

Diarrhea or constipation

Dry mouth

Increased sweating

Headaches

Jitteriness or agitation

Although a tremendous amount of research has demonstrated the efficacy of antidepressants for people who have unipolar (nonbipolar) depression, there actually are few investigations of the use of these medications, particularly the newer ones, in bipolar individuals. There are, however, two very recent large-scale studies that I'd like to mention because I think the findings are particularly important.

The first study was conducted to determine whether antidepressants add to the efficacy of mood stabilizers in bipolar depression. Study participants were assigned randomly to receive either an antidepressant or a pill placebo in addition to their mood stabilizer (which they already were maintained on) for the 6-month period of the investigation. Results showed that the two groups did not differ in outcome—there was no advantage to taking antidepressants.

Another recent study showed more promising results for the use of antidepressants. In this investigation people with bipolar depression received one of two atypical antipsychotics (because of their mood-stabilizing properties)—Zyprexa or Seroquel—either alone or in combination with an SSRI antidepressant, Prozac. Although Zyprexa and Seroquel alone were both effective, findings revealed that the combination of Zyprexa and Prozac yielded even better results. In fact, at least partly because of the results of this study the two drugs have been combined into one substance (brand name **Symbyax**), now available as one of only two FDA-approved treatments for bipolar depression (see the sidebar on page 109).

Antidepressants

Brand name	Pharmaceutical name
SSRIs	
Celexa	citalopram
Lexapro	escitalopram
Luvox	fluvoxamine
Paxil	paroxetine
Prozac	fluoxetine
Zoloft	sertraline
Atypical antidepressants	
Desyrel	trazodone
Remeron	mirtazapine
—	nefazodone
Wellbutrin	bupropion
Tricyclics	
Anafranil	clomipramine
Ascendin	amoxapine
Elavil	amitriptyline
Ludiomil	maprotiline
Norpramine	desipramine
Pamelor	nortriptyline
Tofranil	imipramine
Vivactil	protriptyline
MAOIs	
Eldepryl	selegiline
Emsam	selegiline transdermal system
Marplan	isocarboxazid
Nardil	phenelzine
Parnate	tranylcypromine
SSNRIs	
Cymbalta	duloxetine
Effexor	venlafaxine
Pristiq	desvenlafaxine
Combination drugs	
Symbyax	fluoxetine and olanzapine

What You Need to Know about Benzodiazepines

- Used short term in high doses for hyperactivity/agitation in acute mania.
- Used for insomnia.
- Used to treat coexisting anxiety symptoms.
- High potential for addiction.
- Risk of respiratory depression and death if combined with other drugs, such as sedatives, narcotics, and alcohol.

Benzodiazepines

The class of drugs known as benzodiazepines, also referred to as "minor tranquilizers," has three uses in the treatment of bipolar disorder: as a short-term intervention for acute mania in those who are hyperactive or agitated, to treat co-occurring anxiety disorders or prominent anxiety symptoms, and for insomnia. Although the medications are very effective sedatives, they generally are used judiciously because they have a high potential for addiction. Also, benzodiazepines may not be

FDA-Approved for the Treatment of Bipolar Disorder

Acute mania	Acute depression	Maintenance (preventing or delaying recurrences)
Lithium	Symbyax	Lithium
Depakote	Seroquel	Lamictal
Tegretol		Zyprexa
Zyprexa		Abilify
Risperdal		
Seroquel		
Geodon		
Abilify		

appropriate if your partner is experiencing depression, as the drugs are central nervous system depressants.

The medications that fall into this group of drugs include **Ativan** (lorazepam), **Klonopin** (clonazepam), **Librium** (chlordiazepoxide), **Tranxene** (clorazepate), **Valium** (diazepam), and **Xanax** (alprazolam). Some, like Ativan and Xanax, are shorter acting, while others, like Klonopin, are longer acting (the shorter-acting benzodiazepines are thought to have a higher potential for addiction). Common side effects of these drugs include sedation, sleepiness, feeling slowed down, decreased coordination, and memory loss.

Because these drugs are central nervous system depressants, they should not be taken with alcohol (which also is a central nervous system depressant) or other sedative medications. In addition, because of their potential for lethality in large doses, these drugs should be given only in limited quantities to individuals considered to be at risk for suicide.

Other Medical Treatments You Should Know About

There are several medical treatments, some of which have been around for decades and others that are much newer, that may be used as alternatives or adjuncts to standard pharmacological treatment for bipolar disorder.

Electroconvulsive Therapy (ECT)

Unfortunately, because of how it's often referred to ("shock therapy") and portrayed by the media, as well as the overuse of this procedure when it first became available, ECT has gotten an unfavorable reputation. The truth of the matter is that ECT is a highly effective treatment for severe, acute manic, mixed, and depressed states, particularly for those who have not responded sufficiently to medications (for this reason, it's often considered "the treatment of last resort"). Another benefit of the treatment is that it can be administered safely during pregnancy.

Today ECT is done under general anesthesia. The procedure takes a matter of minutes (most of the time is spent putting the person under and the person then coming out of anesthesia) and involves delivering just a couple of seconds of electrical stimulation to the brain, through electrode disks applied to the head. The electrical stimulus produces a "seizure," but one that is without the jerking movements usually associated with true seizures.

ECT usually is conducted intensively—often three times a week—in a series of 6 to 12 treatments for the acute treatment of a mood episode, and then followed with "maintenance therapy," where the frequency of treatments decreases to every few weeks or even months. The treatment can be administered on an inpatient basis for those who are hospitalized or on an outpatient basis.

A common side effect of ECT is memory loss—approximately two-thirds of people receiving the treatment say it affects their memory in some way. Many have trouble remembering events that occur during the 2 to 4 weeks that they receive intensive treatment. Some report losing memories of events that occurred during the period just before treatment; still others have memory lapses for isolated situations from their pasts.

Depressed bipolar individuals who receive ECT can become hypomanic (they are less likely to develop full-blown mania). But unlike antidepressant medications, the treatment has not been shown to increase mood cycling.

Rapid Transcranial Magnetic Stimulation (rTMS)

Recently developed as an alternative to ECT, rTMS is a way of stimulating the brain that does not induce "seizure" activity and does not require anesthesia. The technique relies on the principle of electromagnetism. A magnetic coil is held against the scalp, and the magnetic field created by the coil induces a very small electrical current in the brain. (The procedure is also unlike ECT in that no electricity passes through the skull.)

Preliminary findings are promising—they suggest that this treatment may be effective for both depression and mania without causing the memory problems associated with ECT. However, since the procedure (and the research conducted on it) still is very much in its infancy, the availability of this treatment is limited, though something to look forward to on the horizon.

Vagus Nerve Stimulation (VNS)

A very recent procedure for treatment-resistant depression, VNS involves implanting under the skin a device that delivers electrical stimulation to the vagus nerve. Although the treatment was originally developed for epilepsy, the discovery of its mood-enhancing effects led to research into its efficacy in alleviating depression. To date (as of the time of this writing) research has produced mixed results: some studies have found a definite superior effect for the treatment while others have had less impressive results. However, if your partner has not responded to other treatments for bipolar depression, it may behoove the two of you to look into the latest findings on VNS (research conducted during the past 2 years, that is, since the writing of this book) by conducting a search on the Internet. You can also look on the website of Cyberonics, the company that is marketing the VNS device that has been approved by the FDA for treatment-resistant depression.

Phototherapy

As I mentioned briefly in Chapter 2, people who have a seasonal pattern to their mood episodes—specifically wintertime depressions—often benefit from increasing their exposure to light. Phototherapy involves full-spectrum white, bright light exposure, aimed directly onto the eyes using a light box or light visor as the source of illumination (the light box requires the individual to sit still in front of it, whereas the visor allows for movement).

Phototherapy sessions usually are conducted in the morning for anywhere from 30 minutes to 2 hours, the amount of time depending on the strength of the light source, the severity of the depressive symptoms, and the speed of the response. Although the treatment appears to be highly and rapidly effective, there is a risk of initiating switches into mania or hypomania as there is with many other treatments for bipolar depression.

Although initial studies included only individuals with seasonal symptom patterns, recent research suggests that phototherapy may be as effective for depressions that do not follow a seasonal pattern. Also, while the procedure has been shown to work by itself alone, it may be even more efficacious when combined with medication.

Thyroid Augmentation

Research indicates that 30 to 50% of people who do not have a complete alleviation of their depressions from traditional psychiatric drugs benefit from increasing their levels of T3 (the active form of thyroid hormone) with the prescription medication Cytomel, even if they do not test positive for hypothyroidism. Rapid cyclers and women are most likely to benefit from thyroid augmentation. Supplemental thyroid hormone tends to have few side effects, but some people complain of feeling anxious or "racy," in which case the dose of medication can be reduced.

Sleep Deprivation

Interestingly, research has shown consistently that depressed patients—including those with bipolar depression—experience an improvement in mood following a night of missing sleep. Unfortunately, this effect diminishes for most after getting normal sleep the next night. As a result, various studies have looked at a number of ways to try to maintain the initial antidepressant effect of sleep deprivation. Results have shown that alternating repeated sleep deprivation—that is, 3 days without sleep—with 3 days of sleep, has some sustained benefit. The use of adjunct medication has also been shown to prevent the rapid relapse into depression typically seen following cessation of sleep deprivation treatment.

Unfortunately, outside of the scientist's laboratory sleep deprivation as a treatment for depression is still considered controversial. In addition to the questionable ethical and pragmatic issues involved in keeping patients up at night, the procedure carries the risk (in some studies, apparently a very high risk) of switching people into mania or hypomania. Given all of these considerations, *the treatment should be done only under the close supervision of a doctor who has prescribed it.*

What Therapy Can Do for Your Partner and You

Because bipolar disorder is largely genetic and thought to be caused by chemical imbalances in the brain, for many years psychologists and other nonphysician mental health professionals were considered to have very limited roles in the treatment of the disorder. Primarily they were relegated to providing emotional support and assisting in fostering medication compliance. Recent scientific studies, however, have demonstrated powerful effects for "skills-oriented" psychological therapies. These treatments, when administered in conjunction with psychiatric drugs, have been shown to work faster and keep people well longer than medication alone or medication used together with more traditional, generic "talk therapy."

These days most doctoral-level (PhD or PsyD) clinical psychologists are trained to do skills-oriented treatments. Generally, these therapists undergo a 5-year postcollege graduate school program that includes a 1-year internship. Other types of mental health professionals with less extensive training may, however, have the competence to provide therapy to your partner, including master's level psychologists, clinical or psychiatric social workers, and marriage and family therapists. (In most states only psychologists can refer to themselves as such; individuals with other types of degrees may call themselves, for example, "therapists" or "counselors" or "psychotherapists," but not "psychologists.") Also, as I mentioned earlier in this chapter, some psychiatrists—though relatively few these days—conduct therapy. However, generally (and I do mean generally) speaking, the type of therapy offered by medical doctors rarely is the skills-oriented approach that's been found most helpful for bipolar disorder.

Cognitive-Behavioral Therapy (CBT)

CBT is a marriage of cognitive therapy and behavior therapy, or behavior modification. This mode of treatment is based on the idea that certain unhelpful types of thoughts and behaviors can trigger, escalate, and lengthen mood episodes. CBT has been used extensively with many psychiatric disorders, including unipolar depression, but its application to bipolar disorder is more recent. Also, although there are many different forms of CBT, including the one I use, they share the same general focus on the interplay among thoughts, behaviors, and emotions.

CBT sessions usually are conducted individually, weekly, but in some cases a group format is used. It is a time-limited treatment, like most skills-oriented therapies, that generally spans 6 months (although periodic "booster sessions" may be provided on a less intensive basis thereafter). The best time to begin CBT is when your partner has been stabilized on his medication, although the treatment can be adapted for use during an episode of illness.

The cognitive component of CBT helps people learn how to identify and then challenge (and ultimately change) their unhelpful, distorted thoughts and beliefs. For example, extremely pessimistic or negative ways of looking at things—"I'm a failure," "Nothing will ever work out for me"—can trigger or accompany (and worsen) depression. At the other extreme people who are manic or hypomanic tend to view themselves, the world, and their future in an overpositive or unduly optimistic way. A manic (or hypomanic) person may think, "I'm lucky, everything's going my way," or that she is powerful or invincible. These distortions in thinking can lead to bad judgments and risk-taking behavior that results in painful consequences. In CBT sessions the therapist points out and challenges these distorted ways of looking at things. For example, if your partner made a global negative statement about herself, the therapist would question the generalization by coming up with—together with your partner—evidence that contradicts the belief. If your partner demonstrates denial or minimization of the illness, saying things like "It's no big deal that I have bipolar disorder" or "I'm doing better so I don't need medication anymore" (see Chapter 3 for more on denial), the therapist will address these attitudes too.

In between sessions people monitor their thoughts—actually write them down on forms designed for this purpose—and then examine them for illogic or bias, which they then counter with a more rational, alternative thought or series of thoughts. Through continued practice, your partner would eventually become skilled at changing unhelpful automatic thoughts into more reasonable and helpful ones. The ultimate goal is for the new rational thoughts to become habitual and essentially replace the old irrational thinking style.

The behavioral component of CBT can contain a number of techniques that can be useful to those with bipolar disorder. Generally, early in treatment, education about bipolar illness is presented and issues surrounding medication compliance are addressed. People also monitor their moods every day (using a standardized scale and records that are supplied for this purpose) and learn to be vigilant for their own idiosyncratic early warning signs of mood episodes. Other important components of the behavioral aspect of treatment include making lifestyle modifications, such as maintaining good sleep hygiene and keeping a regular routine or daily schedule (scheduling activities, including pleasant ones, and monitoring stimulation levels), and identifying and controlling (or at least minimizing) cues and triggers of mood episodes.

Because stress and anxiety frequently trigger mood episodes, during CBT your partner also may:

- Learn strategies for *problem solving and decision making*.
- Work on enhancing *interpersonal communication* skills to reduce relationship conflicts.
- Learn general *stress management* skills, like relaxation techniques or meditation.
- Overcome fears and phobias (if present) with *exposure-based procedures*.

At the time of this writing, six studies had been published that investigated the effectiveness of CBT for bipolar disorder. Five of the six showed that CBT, when administered along with medication, produced better outcomes than medication alone or medication plus non-skills-oriented psychotherapy. (In the one study that did not find an overall advantage for CBT, a subset of participants—individuals who had no more than 12 lifetime episodes of illness—showed significant therapeutic effects from CBT. Individuals who had a more highly recurrent form of illness—more than 12 lifetime episodes—actually got *worse*.) Of note, four of the studies conducted included people who had bipolar II disorder, in addition to individuals with bipolar I disorder.

On the basis of the available data and my own professional and personal experience, I would recommend CBT for people who are relatively stable following an episode of illness or experiencing some residual mood symptoms, but preferably not in the midst of a major mood episode. The treatment also seems best for those who are fairly verbal and have a certain level of insight—that is, they can reflect about their disorders—and for people who are reasonably committed and motivated to participate in treatment since a fair amount of "homework" has to be done between sessions. But even those who are more severely disturbed and/or lower functioning can benefit from some of the more basic behavioral elements of the treatment—like psychoeducation, lifestyle changes, and mood monitoring.

While it's not that difficult to find an experienced cognitive–behavioral therapist, it may be more complicated to locate one who has expertise in using this treatment with bipolar disorder. One way you and your partner can start is by contacting the Massachusetts General Hospital Bipolar Clinic in Boston (the clinic uses CBT in its program). Another avenue is to search the Web for individual practitioners of CBT and examine their credentials. Also, some CBT professional associations have referral lists for potential consumers (like the Association for Behavioral and Cognitive Therapies, the Academy of Cognitive Therapy, and the American Academy of Cognitive and Behavioral Psychology).

Dialectical Behavior Therapy (DBT)

DBT originally was developed for the treatment of borderline personality disorder. But because bipolar disorder shares some of the key features of borderline personality disorder—including emotional regulation problems and self-injurious and other high-risk behaviors—and some people have both disorders, the treatment is now being used increasingly for those with bipolar disorder, both by individual practitioners and at bipolar disorder clinics at major medical centers throughout the United States (including, for example, the Stanford School of Medicine and the Mount Sinai Medical Center in New York). The treatment uses some of the same methods for change that are part of traditional CBT, but also includes a focus on "acceptance"—teaching the bipolar person how to accept emotional states and circumstances that can't immediately be changed. (The concept of acceptance also extends to the therapist's validation of the individual's experience.)

The treatment consists of both individual and group therapies, usually conducted over the course of 1 year. Weekly individual psychotherapy sessions target problematic events or behaviors from the previous week, focusing on alternatives the person could have used to better manage the situations. In addition to the scheduled in-person sessions, phone contact with the individual therapist between visits is a part of DBT. The therapy also promotes the use of skills acquired from the group therapy (see below).

The group therapy also is conducted weekly, with sessions lasting from 2 to 2½ hours. (Typically, a therapist other than the one who is conducting the individual psychotherapy conducts the group therapy,

and therapist consultation—the individual and group therapists interacting on a regular basis—is considered another key component of this
treatment). The sessions consist of teaching group members four different sets of skills: (1) core mindfulness, (2) interpersonal effectiveness, (3) emotional regulation, and (4) distress tolerance.

Core mindfulness skills are derived from Buddhist meditation
practices and are used to help people become aware of the different
aspects of an experience and to develop the ability to stay with the
experience in the present moment. Interpersonal effectiveness skills
focus on teaching effective ways to achieve one's goals with other
people: how to ask for what one needs, how to say "no" effectively,
and how to form and maintain healthy relationships with others. With
emotional regulation skills participants learn ways of altering or modu-
lating distressing emotional states, like anger, anxiety, and depression.
Finally, distress tolerance teaches individuals how to live through, and
find meaning in, disturbing situations that cause emotional pain.

Although there has been considerable research on the use of this
treatment for borderline personality disorder, at the time of this writing there have been only two reported studies—one with adolescents
and one with adults—that included bipolar individuals. In both, when
participants' outcomes were compared to their status before treatment,
findings showed significant improvement as a result of treatment. However, both of the two investigations were "uncontrolled" (there were
no comparison groups receiving alternative or placebo treatments), so
these data should be considered very preliminary at best.

Clinically speaking, though, on the face of it I would think this
mode of treatment would be particularly beneficial for bipolar people
who are not currently in a major, full-blown mood episode, but either
have some residual symptoms from a recent mood episode or are relatively stabilized. The treatment focuses a lot of attention on methods
for eliminating impulsive mood-dependent high-risk behaviors, so if
your loved one has a history of suicidal thoughts and/or behaviors or
other types of self-harm (for example, substance abuse or binge eating), or acts out during hypomanic or manic episodes (excessive gambling or shopping, sexual infidelity), this treatment may be particularly beneficial. In addition, people who have co-occurring borderline
personality disorder or anxiety disorders could benefit from different
aspects of the skills modules for these problems, as well as for their
bipolar illness.

If your partner is interested in receiving DBT treatment and is not near the clinic in California mentioned earlier or the one in New York, I recommend calling the University of Washington in Seattle's DBT center (the originator of this treatment approach is on the faculty there). This facility may be able to refer you to someone in your area who is trained in DBT. Another alternative is to do a search on the Internet—there are many sites of individual DBT practitioners and of organizations that have referral lists of DBT providers. Also, the Behavioral Tech, LLC, website (*behavioraltech.org*) has a link to a DBT therapist directory.

Interpersonal and Social Rhythm Therapy (IPSRT)

IPSRT is a treatment that incorporates interpersonal psychotherapy—a therapy that was developed for helping individuals with depression resolve relationship difficulties—with techniques that focus on stabilizing daily routines or "rhythms." It was developed specifically for the treatment of bipolar disorder. The theory behind the therapy stems in large part from the notion that disrupted body rhythms (resulting from both conflicted relationships and other stresses and disturbed biological functions like the sleep–wake cycle) contribute to the onset of bipolar mood episodes.

To help stabilize their daily routines, people are asked to record their mood states and events and activities (including such things as what time they eat dinner, which TV shows they watch at night, what time they go to sleep) and level of social stimulation (the amount of "high" versus "low" intensity contact—for example, going to a party or family gathering versus making a telephone call to schedule a haircut) each day on a "social rhythm" chart.

The interpersonal component of the treatment has individuals identify and then resolve key relationship problems. People develop an "interpersonal inventory" of their social networks, including all current and potential conflicts and stresses that may upset their emotional stability. The therapist then works with the individual to develop methods for reducing the conflicts and, in so doing, helps stabilize that person's daily social rhythms.

In one large study with acutely ill bipolar patients, researchers found that those receiving IPSRT, in conjunction with medication, had a better 2-year outcome than individuals who received an intensive psychoeducational therapy. In the recent multisite study on the treatment of bipolar disorder, IPSRT was found to be as effective as CBT and family-focused therapy (FFT, discussed next).

One of the advantages of this treatment approach is that it apparently can be used effectively when someone with a bipolar I disorder is in a full-blown mood episode. It does, however, involve a fair amount of charting, making it an "active" as opposed to a more "passive" mode of treatment, so I would think that the bipolar person would need a reasonable amount of motivation to benefit. This type of treatment also would be particularly helpful to those who have significant sleep–wake disturbances (very common among bipolar people and shown to have a significant association with episode recurrence) and/or recurrent conflict in their interpersonal relationships, including with their partners. (Remember, though, that IPSRT is an individual treatment, so when key relationships are targeted for improvement, this occurs without the spouse or partner of the ill person present.)

If your partner is interested in locating a therapist who conducts this type of treatment, a good way to start is by calling the Bipolar Disorders Clinic at the University of Pittsburgh School of Medicine (the originator of IPSRT is on the faculty there).

Family-Focused Therapy (FFT)

FFT is a modified version of a treatment that focused on how family dynamics and relationships can contribute to the wellness or illness of a person with a major psychiatric disorder. It was originally designed to strengthen social support and reduce "expressed emotion," that is, critical, hostile, or overinvolved attitudes and behaviors that family members may exhibit toward the ill individual, and it's been adapted specifically for use with people who have bipolar disorder and their spouses/partners or other close family members. Unlike the other psychosocial treatments described in this chapter, FFT sessions will include both you and your partner, who will both be required to sign informed-consent forms to participate. The treatment typically is administered over a 9-month period.

The heart of the therapy is educational. During the early stages of treatment your family learns about bipolar symptoms, etiology, course and prognosis, and treatment. You also learn about self-management of the illness, including how to detect early warning signs of a possible recurrence and develop an action plan (such as when to call the doctor) for handling a recurrence. Methods for dealing with medication compliance also are addressed.

Later on in the treatment you and your partner work on communication and problem-solving skills. The therapist also will teach your family four basic communication skills: how to express positive feelings, how to express negative feelings, active listening, and how to make requests for change. Problem-solving techniques are applied to family problems that are common in bipolar disorder.

Several studies have examined the effectiveness of FFT. The first two showed that when the treatment was combined with medication bipolar individuals had a better outcome over a 1- to 2-year period following an episode than they did on medication alone or on medication and supportive individual therapy. Recent results from a large-scale multisite investigation of the treatment of bipolar disorder showed that FFT was as effective as other skills-oriented therapies, including CBT and IPSRT.

Most of the research on FFT included the families of people with bipolar I disorder. My own appraisal of this form of therapy is that it probably works best when the bipolar disorder is relatively severe (like bipolar I disorder) and/or your partner is lower functioning.

Goals of Skills-Oriented Therapies

- Educate about bipolar disorder and help the individual accept having the illness.
- Identify early warning signs of mood episodes.
- Develop strategies for solving problems and dealing with interpersonal conflicts.
- Learn stress management techniques to keep anxiety to a minimum.
- Develop lifestyle changes and coping skills that promote good mood health.
- Promote medication compliance.
- Offer a source of emotional support.
- Be an avenue for including family members in the treatment process.

A Comparison of Four Skills-Oriented Therapies

	CBT	DBT	IPSRT	FFT
Psychoeducation	+++	+	+	+++
Medication compliance	+++	+	+	+++
Reducing high-risk behavior	++	+++	+	++
Interpersonal skills	+++	+++	+++	+++
Stress reduction techniques	+++	++	+++	+
Problem-solving skills	+++	+++	++	+++
Stabilize daily routine and sleep–wake cycle	++	+	+++	++
Detecting early warning signs	+++	+	+	+++
Family attends sessions	*	*	*	+++
Group (nonfamily) sessions	*	+++	—	—

+   Is a minor component of the treatment.

++   Is a moderate component of the treatment.

+++   Is a major component of the treatment.

—   Not applicable.

*   Varies according to the individual therapist.

Higher-functioning people may find the inclusion of their significant other in all sessions intrusive and feel that their individual needs and issues are being sacrificed to the family focus. But FFT may be just the right treatment if you and your partner are embroiled in conflict over the manifestations of the disorder or you have to play a caregiver role because your loved one's illness is very severe. This therapy is also a good choice if you have children who are being affected by the disorder.

Of note, the Beth Israel Medical Center in New York offers a "family-inclusive treatment" that includes many of the components of standard FFT. Another avenue for finding a FFT therapist is to contact the University of Colorado's psychology department (the originator of FFT is on the faculty there).

Self-Help and Support Groups

Before leaving the subject of psychotherapy, I want to briefly mention two other sources of emotional support—one for your bipolar partner and one for you. Bipolar *self-help groups* can be very useful as an adjunct to skills-oriented psychological treatments (particularly those that are not conducted in groups) because they offer individuals a chance to interact with other people who are experiencing similar problems. Sometimes groups are run by one or more group members, while in other cases a mental health professional serves as the leader of the group (if the meeting is run by a mental health professional, there may be a nominal fee rather than being free of charge). Some meetings are "open," which means that your loved one can, if desired, take you along.

For the family members of individuals with bipolar disorder, *family support groups* are a place to interact with other partners of bipolar people. A group like this can help you feel less alone in your situation. Because these groups often are supported by national organizations, participation also can be a way of getting up-to-date information on bipolar illness. Usually, family support groups are free of charge. Many are open to people who have the illness as well as their family members, so if your mate is uncomfortable with the idea of your going to a group like this, you might want to suggest that he come with you. See the Resources section for a list of organizations that offer self-help and family support groups.

Knowledge is certainly power, and I hope the information about treatment options in this chapter has given you confidence that real help is available. But now that you know that the professionals have treatments that are effective, you need to figure out the tricky balancing act of defining your own role in the treatment process. How involved can and should you be in your partner's care? How can you respect important boundaries—yours and your partner's? How much help can you give without cultivating helplessness in your mate, or helping so much that you're left depleted? The next chapter will help you figure out how to contribute to your partner's well-being without sacrificing your own.

5

You, Your Loved One, and the Doctors

The Team Approach to Getting and Staying Well

Dianne's fiancé, Patrick, has stopped taking his medication again. A science fiction author, he says the mood stabilizer hampers his creativity and makes it difficult for him to work. But Dianne sees that Patrick already is hypomanic—very irritable, working 12 to 14 hours a day, hardly sleeping at night, and talking a lot at a very fast pace—and fears he's headed for another full-blown manic episode.

Dianne: *Patrick, you have to go back on your medication.*

Patrick: *I can't take that stuff. It messes up my ability to work.*

Dianne: *Babe, I know it's difficult for you to write when you're on the medicine, but you know it's completely impossible when you get manic. Your ideas get "very loose" and unfocused—you've said you can't use anything you write during those times.*

Patrick: *But it will be different this time—you'll see—I'll keep things under control; I won't become manic.*

Dianne: *That's what you said the last time you stopped the medication.*

Patrick: *But I just can't live this way, not being able to keep a thought in my head!*

Dianne: *You can't live off the medication! Stopping the medication always ends in disaster! Remember when you took a swing at that guy in the movie theater? How about when you got the DUI and had to spend the night in jail? And what about our former best friends, Carol and John, whom you offended the last time you had an episode?*

Patrick: *Okay, the episodes are a problem, but I'm not getting manic this time.*

Dianne: *Look at your sleep—that's a sure sign that you're getting up there. And all the hours you're working, another clear sign.*

Patrick: *I'm just being productive.*

Dianne: *But you always get "productive" right before you get manic. Think back to last summer. Do you remember what happened?*

Patrick: *Um ... yeah, I remember.*

Dianne: *So you see that what's going on now is just the beginning?*

Patrick: *It might be.*

Dianne: *It might be?*

Patrick: *Yeah, okay, I see what you're saying, but what do you want me to do? I need to be able to work!*

Dianne: *Why don't we go see your psychiatrist and ask him about other options? Maybe he'll lower your dose, or possibly there's some drug out there that doesn't have the same side effects.*

Patrick: *That's an idea. Maybe I could get by on less medicine or a different drug altogether. They come out with new drugs all the time.*

Dianne: *Right. We'll go together and check it out as soon as he has an appointment available. In the mean-*

> *time, promise me you'll take your medication. I*
> *don't want to see you sick again. Promise me.*

Patrick: *Okay, I'll do it, but just for now. We have to find*
> *a better solution.*

There's no one with a better vantage point than you to see changes—good or bad—that are taking place in your mate. No one, not even the doctor, knows your partner to the extent you do. And given your intimate, emotional connection with your loved one, you're also in a position to influence the choices your mate makes in how he manages his illness day to day and to assist the doctors in achieving their goals. That's why you can be such an important part of your loved one's "treatment team," the group of individuals who share the common goal of promoting your mate's mental health.

In any "team," each individual has a distinct role to play. Your role may include:

- *Learning about bipolar disorder* so you can understand the nature of your partner's illness and the different treatment options available
- *Staying in contact with your loved one's doctors* so you can be aware of and support your mate's treatment
- *Knowing your mate's early warning signs* of mania and depression so you can assist your partner and the doctors in identifying potential mood episodes before they get out of hand
- *Taking care of yourself* by setting personal boundaries, putting aside time just for you, and, possibly, joining a support group or entering therapy to help you cope with your mate's illness

That last item is often the most important one. That's because being a helpful member of your partner's treatment team also means knowing what *not* to take on. As one example, your position does not include making treatment decisions. That is, of course, the domain of the doctors, the mental health professionals who are trained to treat bipolar illness. It also doesn't mean that you take responsibility for your partner's mental health—in the final analysis, it's really your mate's job to take care of himself. Your role also doesn't include being available without limits. Ignoring your own needs and overall well-being not only diminishes you as an individual—both in and outside of your relationship—but ultimately will affect what you have to offer to your spouse. In other words, if you don't take care of you, there eventually won't be much of a "you" left to give.

Taking the time to read this book can say a lot of different things about you. Certainly it suggests you want to better understand your mate's illness. For many of you, it shows you need some support and guidance to help you cope with having a bipolar partner. It may also indicate an interest in learning how you can play an active role in helping your partner attain mood stability. In this case, like in Dianne's, there are many ways you can contribute to this end: by being a good observer, providing feedback to your partner when appropriate, and reinforcing and supporting the efforts your teammates—your partner and the professionals—put forth.

Together all of you—you, your partner, and the doctors—can, if you so choose, work together to create a force that will give bipolar disorder a run for its money, a force to be reckoned with. How does this process begin? The very first step is to meet with your loved one's doctors.

Meeting with Your Partner's Doctors

The extent to which you'll need to be involved with your partner's doctors depends to a large degree on the severity of your mate's illness and her response to treatment. For example, if your mate becomes psychotic, violent, suicidal, or otherwise out of control during mood episodes, you'll have to be in contact with the mental health professionals providing her care at those times. But if your partner has a mild form of bipolar disorder that is well controlled, you may never *need* to be in direct contact with your loved one's doctors. Still, communicating with your partner's mental health professionals is always a very good idea for all of these reasons:

• *Doctors value information provided by people close to their patients.* In fact, you may be better able to describe mood-related behaviors—more objectively and with more clarity—than your mate can (your mate, on the other hand, is the one who best can describe his own internal state—that is, thoughts and feelings). Also, given your emotional and physical proximity to your spouse, you are in a position to see subtle shifts in your partner's mood and behavior that the doctor isn't privy to.

• *It keeps you abreast of your loved one's treatment plan.* Since medication noncompliance is such a common occurrence among bipolar people (see Chapter 6), you want to be aware of the specific medications, including their doses, the doctor is prescribing. You also want to know when your loved one is starting a new medication so you can help monitor for adverse reactions (see Chapter 4).

• *It's a way of supporting your loved one and showing you care.* Going with your partner to doctor visits in general (with your mate's permission) shows that you care about your loved one's health and well-being. It also helps prevent your spouse from feeling alone in the treatment process, that she has someone to share the experience with.

• *It reinforces the treatment team concept.* In other words, it shows that you, your loved one, and the doctor are all working together toward a common goal: your partner's mental health.

• *It lays the groundwork you'll need in the event of an emergency.* It's important to have a connection established in case your partner takes a turn for the worse. In an emergency situation, when you are flooded with emotions, it's easier to reach out to someone you already have a relationship with rather than a stranger.

It's been my experience that most psychiatrists and psychologists welcome the input of the significant others when treating bipolar individuals. For example, they usually are very open to conducting joint sessions. You should know, though, that some doctors will not be willing to communicate with you—in person or possibly even on the phone—without your partner present, or they may be willing to do so only if they have a release signed by your mate that authorizes them to share information with you.

Some people who have no prior exposure to mental health professionals are intimidated by the idea of speaking with one. They are afraid they will themselves come under scrutiny. (I can't tell you how many times individuals I meet outside my work ask me, "Are you analyzing me?" and other questions like this when they find out I'm a psychologist.) It may be helpful to keep in mind that, in all likelihood, your partner's psychiatrist or psychologist is interested in you solely

What If Your Partner Doesn't Want to Authorize the Doctor to Share Information with You?

The spouse of a patient of mine came up with an interesting way around this. He sent a detailed letter to his mate's psychiatrist to make sure the doctor was aware of certain things that he was concerned the physician might not already know. Since the communication was one-way, there was no need for the doctor to have a signed release.

in relation to your spouse and not you as a separate person. When it comes to their work, doctors are focused on their patients: they're not in the habit of providing services (an "analysis" or what have you) to those who aren't under their care.

But what about your loved one's comfort with your being in the room? Will your partner be okay with it? Chances are he will. In fact, people who have this illness often take their partners with them to appointments on their own initiative. In my own practice, if I find that a new patient wants to bring his partner with him to the first session, the couple generally is there for one of two reasons: bipolar disorder or couple therapy (or both).

But what if your partner doesn't feel this way? What if your mate feels that your presence would infringe on her privacy, that there are things she wants to be able to say to the doctor without your being there to hear them (such as issues regarding you or your relationship)? If this is the case, you may want to suggest that you split the session in half—that you join your mate for the first part of the visit and then leave for the latter part so she can discuss in confidence whatever needs to be talked about.

Maybe your mate's concern is that you'll report things to the doctor that he doesn't want the doctor to know about (for example, sensitive issues like alcohol consumption, sexual behavior, suicidal thoughts). Handling this can be a bit sticky. On the one hand, you don't want to betray your spouse's trust in you. On the other, secrets really shouldn't be kept from the doctor about things that are relevant to your mate's condition. You'll probably need to figure this one out on the basis of what it is your partner wants to keep from the doctor. If, for instance, your partner doesn't want the doctor to know about something relatively minor (in terms of his mental health problems), I'd let it go. But if your partner wants to keep major signs of mood episodes—like suicidal thoughts, rage episodes, staying in bed, etc.—quiet, you need to have a talk with your mate, perhaps saying something like what Phillip said to Caitlin:

Caitlin: You can go with me to see the doctor as long as you don't tell him about my drinking binge last week. I don't want him to know about it.

Phillip: Caitlin, don't you think it's important for your doctor to know you're mixing alcohol with your medications? Doesn't he also need to know that your drinking is out of control again?

Caitlin: I'm embarrassed about the way I behaved.

Phillip: But he's your doctor. If you can't trust him, then we need to find someone you do trust, because we're counting on this person. He needs to know what's going on.

Caitlin: No, I do trust him. I don't want to find another doctor. We'll tell him. Actually, it probably will be easier to tell him with you there.

Caitlin anticipated that it would be less difficult to share embarrassing information about herself in front of her partner, rather than talking to the doctor alone. Your spouse's willingness to share things like this in front of you will depend to a large extent on the nature of your relationship. If the two of you have very open communication and you are perceived as nonjudgmental, your partner probably will be more comfortable speaking about sensitive topics in your presence. On the other hand, if you are viewed by your mate as critical, she may not want to divulge information of this sort in front of you.

Another reason your partner may not want you to be in the session is that he is concerned that you'll take away from the limited time he has with the doctor. If this is the concern, one way around it is to schedule a double session with the doctor (many doctors will do this) or for your mate to book an additional session without you at another time (possibly later in the week) so he won't feel short-changed.

A variant to this concern is the worry that your being there will be a distraction to the doctor and, as a result, your partner won't get "as good a session" as usual. Unfortunately, there really is no answer to this one other than reiterating the points I went through earlier, the reasons why your at least occasionally meeting with your partner's doctor is so valuable. You might also add that this wouldn't be the first time the doctor has seen a couple (two people at the same time) and that you would think that she (the doctor) would be able to handle this.

If you try to quell your loved one's concerns using the measures I've just outlined but find you're still not getting anywhere, you need to look a little deeper and ask yourself why your partner is so dead set against the idea. We've already discussed the possibility that there's something your spouse's doctor knows about that she doesn't want you to know about, or that there's something you know about that your mate doesn't want the doctor to know about. But a third reason—one we haven't addressed yet—is that by keeping you "out of the loop" your partner may be trying to keep you and your relationship separate from the illness. Even though you may have vowed "for better or for worse, in sickness and in health," your mate may not want you to see the not-so-pretty truth of her condition.

This may strike you as slightly absurd, given that most of you reading this probably are living with the individuals we're talking about. But I can tell you that many years ago I was guilty of trying to shield my husband from knowing too much about my condition. And the reason for this was—as irrational as it may sound—that I was afraid he wouldn't love me anymore, or at least that he wouldn't love me as much, if he knew how "flawed" I was. (Of course, I was wrong. He since knows "the good, the bad, and the ugly," and he's still here 20-plus years later.)

If you suspect that this is the reason your mate doesn't want you involved in the treatment process, think about how you can reassure your loved one about your feelings. Let your mate know, for example, that you're learning all you can about the illness (such as by reading this book) and that you are committed to him and the relationship even in the face of the challenges you know the condition presents. Let your partner know you're there for the long haul, that you can handle this and you have been handling it, that there's no need to hide his inner experiences from you, as awful or terrifying as they may be.

(If you can't actually handle this, see Chapter 10 for more on taking care of yourself.)

I believe the more you reassure your significant other, the more she will open up to you and then be comfortable with your sitting in on her sessions occasionally. But if not, give your loved one some more time and then try again. Sometimes getting a person to agree is just a matter of timing.

Doctor to Doctor: Collaboration between the Professionals

As part of the team concept, it's important that your partner's other health care professionals establish lines of communication with your mate's psychiatrist or whatever physician is managing his psychiatric medication. All of the professionals caring for your partner—and especially those who deliver services that could impact mental health—should interact periodically to make sure they are "on the same page" in their conceptualization and treatment of your mate (this often is referred to as "continuity of care"); this is to make sure they are not inadvertently pursuing goals that are at cross-purposes or overlapping in the services they provide.

If your loved one is seeing a therapist, you and your partner will want to know that there is some form of communication between the therapist and the psychiatrist. Since therapists typically see their patients much more often (usually at least once a week) than psychiatrists do (usually no more than every 1 to 3 months, unless the person is in crisis), they are in a position to see subtle (and sometimes not so subtle) fluctuations in mood that occur over shorter time spans. This information should be shared with the doctor who's prescribing medication so that he has a complete picture of what has occurred between visits. Keep in mind that your mate's physician's ability to do his job well rests very much on the comprehensiveness and quality of the information he has access to. This information can come directly from your partner, from you, and/or from your loved one's therapist.

Some psychiatrists are very open to communicating with psychologists about their mutual patients, while others are not. With any psychiatric disorder, but especially with bipolar disorder, communication and collaboration are really essential to your mate's well-being. In fact, willingness to communicate with me is one criterion I use when deciding whether to refer someone to a particular physician. Even when they're willing, however, I've found some physicians exceptionally hard to get hold of. In these cases, I leave a confidential voice mail message, e-mail, or send a fax with whatever information I feel is important to share.

I remember one case that really highlights the importance of communication between professionals. Twenty-five-year-old Miguel came to see me because he was very depressed—tearful, had lost interest in things, felt hopeless about the future, and was isolating himself from others. Because of his history of previous depressions and the fact that depression runs in his family (I had treated relatives of his in the past), I encouraged him to see Dr. Barnes (not the doctor's real name), one of the psychiatrists I refer to, for a medication evaluation.

The next time I saw Miguel, he had already been to see Dr. Barnes, and he told me the doctor had prescribed an antidepressant for him but he hadn't started taking it yet. In this session, however, Miguel was completely different from how he'd been in the previous session. He continued to say he was depressed but was showing clear signs of mania—couldn't sit still in his chair, was talking a mile a minute, telling me he was drinking to excess and driving while intoxicated and that he had just gone on a buying spree at the local mall, purchasing hundreds of dollars worth of clothing with no idea how he was going to pay for it.

After this visit I called the psychiatrist and told him what I had observed, and we concurred that Miguel probably had bipolar disorder, possibly a rapid-cycling form with mixed symptoms. On the basis of this new information, Dr. Barnes called Miguel and told him not to take the antidepressant, that he was telephoning his pharmacy to prescribe another drug (a mood stabilizer) for him instead.

It's not only therapists and psychiatrists who need to keep the channels of communication open. Other health care professionals too should share with your partner's psychiatrist information that's relevant to your loved one's mental health. For example, since hormones are powerful determinants of mood states, anyone who is being treated by an endocrinologist (or whichever type of physician is treating the hormonal problem) should make sure that copies of his lab results are sent to the psychiatrist.

Your partner's psychiatrist probably will request that basic blood work be done on an annual basis (more often, if your mate is maintained on a medication that requires this; see Chapter 4) unless this is being handled during your spouse's yearly checkup by her primary care physician (internist or family doctor), in which case the findings should be shared with the psychiatrist. On a related note, it's very important that the physician who is prescribing your mate's psychiatric drugs be up-to-date on all other medications that your partner is taking, because of potential drug–drug interactions and also because of the ability of many nonpsychiatric medications to affect mood.

Having Realistic Expectations of Your Partner's Doctor

Bipolar disorder is a serious illness that's not, unfortunately, always easy to get under control. As you have read in the preceding chapter, there are numerous medical and psychological treatments for the disorder, and very often finding the right one or ones—particularly for medications—simply is a matter of trial and error—or, rather, multiple trials and errors.

Jeremy's wife, Suzanne, has been depressed for the past 8 months. Her doctor has tried different combinations of medications but hasn't yet found "a medication cocktail" that completely alleviates her symptoms. But when he finally tried a new approach to bipolar depression—adding thyroid medication (see page 114, Chapter 4) to her drug regimen—the "black veil" that was over Suzanne's head lifted and she was like her old self again.

I know the process of going through different medication trials can be very frustrating and demoralizing—it can be hard to stay upbeat and positive when one drug after the other fails to deliver the hoped-for effect. However, even in the face of the inevitable disappointments, it's important to maintain an optimistic attitude. Otherwise you may end up giving up on finding a solution when an effective treatment is just around the corner.

Even after a person is stabilized on the "right" treatment, factors outside the doctor's control can lead to breakthrough mood episodes. That's what happened to Chris's wife, Bridget.

Although maintained on lithium, and after months of being stable,

Bridget has become manic again. Moving to another city and starting a new job was apparently more than she and the medicine could handle. Chris, though, doesn't exactly see it that way. He thinks Bridget's doctor should have predicted the relapse and done something *before* it happened. "I should report that guy to the medical board for incompetence!" he angrily says under his breath.

No one—including psychiatrists and psychologists—can predict the future. And although stress often precipitates the development of mood episodes, there is no way that Bridget's doctor could have known for sure that this would be the particular outcome in Bridget's case. On the other hand, if the doctor had been aware that Bridget had great difficulty in the past making other moves, he might have made a change in her medication—possibly increasing her lithium—to help prevent her from having a mood episode.

Maybe there were questions the doctor should have asked. Or perhaps Chris, having seen his wife through the other moves, could have shared this information with the doctor. Possibly, close communication between the doctor and Bridget's therapist could have revealed that a big change like relocating was a potential trigger for Bridget. Again, it's impossible to predict the future with 100% certainty, but the more information the treatment team has to work with, the better the odds of heading off mood episodes.

Most doctors do their best to manage bipolar disorder. By "manage" I mean trying to increase *the length of time* between mood episodes; it doesn't mean that your partner won't ever have another episode. Not having additional episodes would mean that your loved one was cured of the illness. And as you know by now, after reading through the previous chapters in this book, bipolar disorder does not, at this point in time, have a cure.

Angela is angry with Dr. Peters because, like the three doctors before him, he hasn't gotten Donald's rapid-cycling under control. Although the medications have lessened Donald's symptoms somewhat, he's virtually never in a state of normal mood. "What's wrong with these psychiatrists?" Angela wants to know. "Don't they know what they're doing?"

Like Chris, Angela is pointing a finger at the medical profession, angry that the doctors haven't been able to "fix" her husband. Unfortunately, the rapid-cycling form of bipolar disorder can be particularly challenging to treat. It's a very disheartening reality of the condition, and I hope in the not too distant future we'll have better means of controlling it. At the time of this writing, however, many people who have this form of bipolar disorder continue to struggle with their illnesses.

It's not just psychiatrists who can have trouble treating bipolar disorder. Therapists run into roadblocks too. For example, it's not uncommon for patients to enjoy their manic or hypomanic highs (despite the potentially catastrophic consequences that can occur) and, consequently, be unwilling to take the steps necessary (like medication adherence and maintaining a normal sleep–wake cycle) to prevent these types of mood episodes from occurring. It's also not unusual for bipolar individuals to view themselves as "victims" of their illnesses, refusing to take personal responsibility for their actions so that change (in therapy) becomes virtually impossible. I'll talk about these and other reasons people sometimes deviate from their treatment in Chapter 6.

Another problem that frequently confronts therapists is the denial that people manifest about their illnesses. Not only does this often occur after the initial diagnosis (as I discussed in Chapter 3) and during the early stages of treatment, but denial can resurface at any point during the course of the illness, even after years of treatment. For example, after 2 years of treatment for his bipolar disorder, Stacy's husband, Terry, suddenly became convinced that there was nothing wrong with him, that he didn't, in fact, have bipolar disorder, and that he should discontinue his medication and also stop therapy with me.

As I'll discuss in the next chapter, it's not uncommon for those with bipolar disorder to think this way after doing well for a sustained period. Because there are no signs of the illness, they conclude either that they never were ill or that the illness has gone away. That's where education about the course of bipolar disorder plays a very important role. Both you and your partner need to understand that the illness is episodic—that there likely will be periods (because of a positive response to treatment or because of the cyclical nature of the disorder) when your mate will be okay. Fortunately, both Stacy and I were able to effectively communicate this to Terry and convince him that he still had bipolar disorder and needed to continue treatment even though he currently was free of mood problems.

Blaming the doctors sometimes is a way of deflecting your own feelings of helplessness and frustration at not being able to do more to

When It's Time to Consider Another Doctor

If the doctor . . .

- *Seems rigid.* Unwilling to deviate from the current treatment plan despite lack of success.
- *Appears rushed.* Doesn't have time for your or your mate's questions or concerns.
- *Seems disinterested* in what you or your mate have to say.
- *Forgets important information,* like treatments that have been tried in the past or details about the current treatment plan.
- *Isn't up-to-date* on new treatments that have become available.
- *Appears insensitive.* Doesn't respond to your partner's distress or makes inappropriate comments.

get your mate well. If you have a tendency to self-blame, externalizing your anger in this way can also be a form of self-protection so that you don't get too down on yourself and even, possibly, depressed.

This is not to say that all doctors are excellent and that you and your partner should not question whether your mate is getting the best possible care. In the sidebar above, I've listed some guidelines you can use to help determine when it may be time to consider changing doctors. However, even if your partner's doctor is doing his best, if he can't get your loved one's illness under control you and your mate still may want to consider getting a second opinion from another physician. Sometimes a fresh perspective is what's needed to turn a difficult-to-treat case into a treatment success.

Having Realistic Expectations of Yourself

Are you constantly exhausted or feeling burned out? Having minor but recurrent physical signs of stress (headaches, stomachaches, back problems, and the like)? Finding your mood isn't as good as it usually is—that you're feeling overwhelmed, anxious, irritable, or down much of the time? Are there changes in your sleep or appetite? Are you and your partner not getting along as well as you used to (for example, you feel resentment toward your partner or the two of you are fighting a lot of the time, or there's a decrease in affectionate and intimate contact)? These can be indications that you've been exceeding the limits of what you can—or should—handle.

Helping your mate without giving away too much of yourself is especially hard for people who have natural caregiving instincts— which is a quality of a many partners of bipolar people—because their tendency is to keep on giving without limits or restrictions. (You may remember years ago when the word *codependent* was very much in vogue. The term actually applies quite nicely here, essentially referring to both the excessive neediness of the caregiver *to be needed* and the insatiable neediness of the care recipient, as well as the unproductive role these two forces can play in a relationship.)

As difficult as it may be, if you're going to keep your own mental and physical health, as well as the health of your relationship, you are going to need to impose limits on what you're willing to do for your mate. The process of setting boundaries may force you to examine certain false beliefs (see the sidebar on the next page) that you hold about your loved one's illness, such as that your loved one's mood swings are somehow your fault or that you can always do something to prevent them (if you were a better husband, wife, lover, partner,

---

Are You Giving Too Much?

- Feeling tired most of the time or burned out
- Recurrent physical signs of stress, like headaches, stomachaches, back pain
- Feeling overwhelmed or anxious
- Irritable much of the time; arguing with your partner or other people
- Feeling down or depressed
- Changes in sleep or appetite
- Angry or resentful toward your mate
- Decreased affection or intimacy in your relationship

Faulty Beliefs

"My partner's illness is my fault."

"I'm responsible for my mate's mental health."

"I can make my spouse well."

"There's nothing I can do at all to improve our lives together."

"The more I give, the better my significant other will be."

"There's not a thing I can do; we're doomed to a terrible future."

your mate wouldn't have mood episodes), or that if you keep on trying you'll be able to "fix" what's "wrong" with your mate, that you'll be able to make him or her well.

Or maybe you are not a natural caregiver and you feel totally outmatched by this challenge. The antidote is not to throw up your hands in surrender but to be proactive, making yourself knowledge-able (which you're already doing by reading this book), and to test out making some small moves that will demonstrate that you do have a certain amount of control—that you can make at least a little differ-ence in your partner's ability to manage the disorder and that there certainly are things you can do to help yourself.

It's important to acknowledge that you are not responsible for your mate's health—that ultimately that is up to her. You can assist, suggest, and support, but you can't live your loved one's life for her. You can offer a certain kind of help, as can your mate's doctors, but at the end of the day it's your loved one who needs to do what has to be done to take care of herself.

How Much Help Is Unhelpful?

In addition to compromising your own emotional and physical well-being and adversely affecting your relationship, providing too much help to your mate can actually backfire, reducing your partner's potential to be well. In other words, your helpfulness may be—without your meaning it to be—unhelpful.

During a period when she was extremely depressed, Barbara had her husband, Jim, help her shower each day. Actually, I shouldn't say that he *helped her* shower because he actually did all of the washing while she stood in the tub. When I found out what was going on, I strongly encouraged Barbara to make a major effort to do this on her own. Jim's bathing her not only was unnecessary, but it fostered Barbara's feelings of helplessness, which in turn further fueled her depression.

Even when they're not having mood episodes, bipolar individuals can be, in a way, very "high maintenance"—they repeatedly impose both large and small demands on their spouses, and when their spouses respond to them *their response* often is to raise the bar even higher. Living with someone like this can make you feel like you have to constantly be "on your toes"—from one "situation" to the next you find yourself trying to fix whatever is awry. But by continually doing this you may be, without meaning to, reinforcing your partner's overreactions and neediness, rather than helping your mate to keep things in perspective and learning to rely on his own resources.

Constantly doing the problem solving for your mate is doing both yourself and your spouse a disservice. When you repeatedly step in, your loved one doesn't use whatever skills she possesses—or develop new ones of her own—and, consequently, she becomes increasingly

Are You Overprotective of Your Partner?

- Do you frequently do things for your mate that he could do for himself?
- Do you make decisions that affect your household without consulting your mate?
- Do you often keep things from your mate because you're concerned that she will get upset?
- When your partner is well, are you uncomfortable with his going places without you or him spending periods of time alone?

dependent and helpless. This, in turn, requires you to be "Johnny on the spot" even more frequently, perpetuating a vicious cycle of giving and taking.

As upsetting as it may be to see your loved one in distress, try to keep in mind that in many cases you will be more helpful to your partner by pulling back and letting your mate navigate whatever problems present themselves. At first it may be difficult for you not to jump in and take over, but after a while it will become more comfortable.

Coping One Day at a Time

It can be incredibly difficult to live with someone who has a chronic illness, and this most certainly is true in the case of bipolar disorder. If you've established a relationship with your partner's doctors, attend a support group, or have a therapist of your own, this is a context in which you can vent your feelings and get support for yourself. As I'll talk about at length in Chapter 10, it's most important that you take time and the measures that will help you cope with the challenges that go along with loving someone who has this disorder.

The mates of people who have bipolar disorder frequently have shared with me the trouble they have dealing with knowing (as you do from Chapter 2) that the course of bipolar illness is recurrent— that people tend to have repeated mood episodes. How, they ask, does one live with the anticipation that his partner will—at some unknown point—become depressed or manic again?

Although there is no easy answer to this question, as I talked about in Chapter 2, I believe the best thing to do is to try your hardest to live in the moment, accepting the present reality as today's truth. Enjoy the good times, the times when your other half is doing well, by experiencing them to their fullest, not by worrying "what if ... ?" and "when will ... ?" That's not to say you shouldn't have a certain level of vigilance, that you should ignore, for example, early warning signs that suggest a mood episode may be on its way or behaviors that make you question whether your mate is taking her medication. But you can't live your life—or at least I don't think you should—filled with fear and trepidation.

I know that this is easier said than done. For most of us living in a Western civilization, it's not our nature to focus on only the present without looking toward the future. This is more of an Eastern philosophical perspective, one often associated with Zen Buddhism. But although foreign to many of us, I believe it's a point of view worth cultivating. You may find that taking meditation classes, reading books on the subject of "mindfulness" (see Resources), or working with a therapist of your own is helpful in achieving this outlook.

As I've discussed in this chapter, because of your emotional and physical proximity to your mate you have the ability to play an important role in your partner's "treatment team," the group of individuals who share the goal of promoting your loved one's mental health. As a team member, however, you need to take care to respect your own, your mate's, and your mate's doctors' limitations and boundaries.

In the next chapter I'll be getting specific about one of the most important things you can do to help your loved one circumvent future mood episodes and achieve mood stability—promoting medication compliance.

10 Steps to Wellness for Your Partner

It's up to your partner to take these steps, but there are ways you can help, described in the following chapters. (And you can benefit from some of the same self-help, such as learning about bipolar disorder and establishing your own social support system; see Chapter 10.)

- Be consistent with treatment—medication; medical and therapy appointments. (Chapter 6)

- Learn about bipolar disorder. (Chapter 7)

- Monitor moods and identify situations that trigger mood fluctuations. (Chapter 7)

- Resolve interpersonal conflicts. (Chapter 7)

- Get sufficient sleep every night. (Chapter 7)

- Keep stress and anxiety low. (Chapter 7)

- Avoid alcohol and street drugs. (Chapter 7)

- Have daily routines. (Chapter 7)

- Have a social support network—family, friends, support group—in place. (Chapter 7)

- Be alert for early warning signs of mood episodes. (Chapters 8 and 9)

6

Helping Your Partner Stick with Medication

During the past couple of weeks Isabel has seen her husband cutting his pills in half. She knows Sam had been taking a whole tablet every night ever since he started the medication, but when she questions him about the change—"Honey, have you reduced your medication?"—he snaps back that he's following his doctor's orders.

Isabel is skeptical. Lately Sam has become increasingly agitated, argumentative, and slightly "paranoid," behaviors that remind her of when he's been manic. Frightened that Sam will continue to get worse, she contacts her husband's doctor to find out for sure what he's supposed to be taking. When the psychiatrist tells her that Sam should be on his maintenance dose of medication—one tablet at bedtime—it is clear that Sam had made the decision to reduce his medication on his own.

"What's the best way to handle this?" Isabel asks herself. "How do I get Sam to own up to what he's been doing and understand the serious consequences that can come from his actions?"

Perhaps you, like Isabel, suspect your partner isn't taking his medications as prescribed and is putting himself at risk for another mood episode. Or maybe you're already seeing symptoms that suggest an episode is on its way.

Medication compliance—or, actually, the lack of it—is a major problem among people with bipolar disorder, possibly more an issue for those with this disorder than for those with any other type of psychiatric illness. In fact, it's more likely than not that at some point during your mate's illness your partner will, on his own, either decrease one or more of his medications or stop taking medication altogether. The problem with this behavior is that it has very serious ramifications for the course of bipolar illness, since *medication inconsistency is the most common cause of new episodes of illness.*

Even mental health professionals who have bipolar disorder—including me—are not immune to this problem. As I've discussed in previous chapters, during my earlier years of treatment I discontinued my medication on a number of occasions. The reasons for stopping were different at different times, as they may be for your loved one as well, but the end result was always the same: I ended up "crashing" and then feeling frantic to get back on the drugs I had forsaken.

You might wonder why anyone would take the risks associated with discontinuing medication in light of the potential—even possibly life-threatening—consequences. Though on the face of it this behavior defies logic, there are a number of possible reasons for it, each of which is listed in the sidebar below and discussed in this chapter.

I'm including a whole separate chapter on the issue of medication adherence before addressing other preventive measures because (1) medication is so critical to bipolar health (as I stressed in Chapter 4, medication is absolutely necessary and the number one component of anyone's treatment), (2) noncompliance is so common, and (3) it can be such a bone of contention between partners.

People may discontinue medication because they ...

- Just don't like the idea of taking drugs.
- Believe that feeling better means they don't need it anymore.
- Don't think it's doing them any good.
- Can't remember to take the medication as prescribed.
- Find the side effects intolerable.
- Miss the "up" times.

"I Don't Like the Idea of Taking Medication"

I don't think anybody with any kind of medical problem relishes the idea of having to take medication. (Well, let me qualify that. I actually have met a few people who are quick to take a drug for whatever ails them, but these individuals are very much in the minority.) For example, I know that my husband does not like taking blood pressure medication, nor does my mother like taking a drug to lower her cholesterol. As I discussed in Chapter 3 when addressing the issue of denial, taking a medication means there's something wrong and, frankly, none of us really wants to think of ourselves that way.

Needing medication also can make people feel vulnerable and dependent, that they can't get by on their own resources, that an outside substance is needed for them to be okay. Many people, too, worry that the medication they take now will, at some point down the road, adversely affect other aspects of their health, like liver functioning (since many drugs are metabolized in the liver).

When it comes to psychiatric illnesses, negative attitudes toward medication often are even stronger. Needing medication to stay physically healthy, such as to prevent life-threatening heart disease, is one thing; needing a drug just to be "normal" can feel like a serious admission of inadequacy or weakness of character because psychiatric disorders still carry a stigma in the minds of many people. People also may be worried that these drugs, because they alter brain chemistry, will change their personalities or have effects on emotions or behavior that feel foreign or uncomfortable or will cause them to "lose control." In addition, because bipolar disorder is essentially a disturbance of mood, some individuals have trouble seeing it as a *medical* problem and, consequently, aren't open to a medical solution. And, of course, rejecting medical treatment for an illness is a way of denying that one has that illness or at least minimizing its significance.

The concept of taking medication regularly makes perfect sense once a person truly acknowledges that bipolar disorder is a lifelong medical illness. But you can see how many preconceived notions—and emotions—your partner might have to break through to get to this point. If your partner is resisting the whole idea of starting regular medication, please go back to Chapter 3 for strategies you can use to help your mate accept the nature of her illness and the need for medication. The exercise that looks at mood disorders in relatives, for example, can help your partner recognize the biological/genetic underpinnings of bipolar disorder, which in turn can make the idea of a medical treatment for the condition more palatable.

Even with considerable effort on your part, however, your loved one may have to learn the hard way how necessary psychiatric drugs are for his condition. I know this can be very tough to observe and frustrating too because from your vantage point the answer to your mate's suffering is so clear. In fact, that's the way Nancy felt about her husband, Lowell, and his repeatedly stopping his medication:

Nancy: I don't understand why you can't see that every time you stop your medication you end up sick again. I feel bad for you, but I'm also angry—angry that you aren't taking care of your problem.

Lowell: I would have been fine if I hadn't lost that account at work. That's what set me back.

Nancy: And 6 months ago? The last time you stopped your medication? What was it then?

Lowell: I can't completely remember, but I think I was stressed out about the stock market. We were losing a lot of money.

Nancy: And the time before that? Last Christmas when you wouldn't leave the bed to watch the kids open their presents?

Lowell: You know that the holidays are always a bad time of year for me.

Nancy: The point is that the medication helps *prevent* you from having reactions like these, even when you're under stress. Why can't you see that?

Lowell: So what do you want me to do? You know I don't want to take it.

Nancy: Make a commitment for 1 year to take all of your medication exactly as the doctor prescribed and let's see what happens. Then we'll know whether what I say is true.

Lowell: There's no way I'm going to commit to a year.

Nancy: Okay, let's do 6 months. That should give us enough time to tell.

Lowell: Okay, okay, I'll try it for 6 months. But if I don't see that things are better, I'm not going to keep taking those pills.

Here Nancy was able to persuade her husband, although certainly not easily, to give the medicine a reasonable trial to see whether it actually made his life better. You can try a similar approach, pointing out to your mate, using specific examples from the past, the relationship between medication discontinuation and mood episodes. Then strongly encourage your partner to test out the "theory" by taking medicine regularly as prescribed for a set period of time and observing the results.

Giving an Ultimatum

Nancy got her husband to agree to consistently take his medication by highlighting instances when the same behavior had been a problem in the past. But what if she hadn't been able to get Lowell to agree to 6 months or any sustained period of time? Should she have considered giving him an ultimatum?

Generally speaking, those with bipolar disorder don't respond well to explicit ultimatums or threats. When cornered they fight back even if it's in their best interest to consider the demand. In other words, to quote a common expression, your partner may respond to an ultimatum by "cutting off his nose to spite his face."

However, if no other strategy has worked and you are at the point where you can't see your relationship continuing because of your partner's lack of treatment adherence, you may choose to go this route. If you do, you are more likely to have success if you present your demand when your partner is not in an angry or irritable frame of mind—for example, not in the middle of an ongoing argument. How you word your demand also is important. Saying, essentially, "Do this or else" is less likely to be effective than an implied demand delivered more tactfully. For example, instead of saying, "Take your medicine or I'm leaving," you might instead say, "I can't continue to live with you off the medication."

Giving an Ultimatum

- Use only as a last resort.
- Word the demand in an implicit, not explicit ("Do this or else"), way.
- Don't use when your partner is in an angry or irritable mood.

Given the effects of his illness on their life together, Nancy might have considered giving Lowell an ultimatum along the lines of "If you want to remain in this relationship with me, you need to take care of your health. I'm not going to stand by and watch you deteriorate—it's not fair to me, it's not fair to you, and it's not fair to our children." Let me emphasize, however, that not only should this approach be used only as a last resort but also that *you really need to mean it.* Generally, you have only one shot at this, and if your spouse finds out you are bluffing—that she can keep living in an irresponsible way and that you won't do anything about it—in all likelihood she will.

"I'm Feeling Better, So I Don't Need It Anymore"

One difficult aspect of having bipolar disorder is recognizing that you still have the illness when you're feeling better. It's not at all unusual for people to have complete "disconnects" about the relationship between the medication they're taking and their freedom from mood swings. For some reason I can't entirely explain (though my guess is it's a form of denial), they simply don't recognize that they're well *because* of the medication; they just think they're well. It's as though they "forget" they have a psychiatric illness. (As you learned in Chapter 2, people also can have well periods between episodes of illness, even if not on medication, which can even further this problem.)

People who have other kinds of psychiatric illnesses typically don't react this way. In fact, those who are being treated for unipolar depression or anxiety disorders, for example, are often reluctant to reduce or discontinue their medication because they fear getting worse. Perhaps because of the overconfidence that comes with mania and hypomania and/or lack of insight into their illness, those with bipolar disorder frequently don't have the same worry about the longevity of their well periods—they assume that they'll be okay even without treatment. That's why it's so important to remind your partner of his previous mood episodes, particularly those that occurred when he wasn't taking medication. Like Nancy, you should try to point out specific time periods (last summer, last Christmas) when your partner had problems. This kind of "in your face" approach forces your partner to recall past mood episodes and makes it very difficult for him to deny having a *recurring* illness or the direct relationship between the recurrences and medication discontinuation.

Kate's medication and therapy with me had paid off: she no longer experienced steep "peaks and valleys" but had achieved good mood stability. Feeling better, she started thinking about pursuing her dream of living in Vermont. She was able to convince her husband that she could handle the change of environment, and they set a date for the move.

When I last saw Kate, it was 2 days before she left for Vermont. She told me she had discontinued her medication a week ago because she felt she wouldn't need it in her new location. She was sure the new environment would be sufficient to keep her well. I voiced my concerns, but she was in no mood to listen—she was hypomanic at the time and completely confident about her decision to stop the medication.

About a month after she left I got a frantic call from Kate's husband. He told me that shortly after they arrived in Vermont Kate's hypomania had worsened dramatically, that she was in a full-blown manic episode and had to be hospitalized.

While certainly the stress of the move could have been a factor in destabilizing this person, stopping her medication didn't help either. Unfortunately, Kate underestimated medication's role in keeping her well and overestimated the positive effect a change of environment would have on her illness. "I'm doing so well I don't need the medication anymore," Kate had said. But she did need her medication. Medication is a major contributor to keeping bipolar disorder under control, and discontinuing it places people at great risk of having new mood episodes.

Significant others—either apart from or together with their mates—also can be lulled into a false sense of security about their partners' illnesses. Seeing your loved one well, you might think she doesn't need as much medication as before or that possibly it could be discontinued altogether. But **please do not suggest a change in how your partner's medication is taken.** Although your observations and input are valuable, your loved one's physician is the only one who is qualified to determine whether the treatment should be changed. So if your partner starts talking about decreasing or stopping her medication, you should strongly urge her to talk over the idea with her doctor rather than make changes on her own.

As I've stressed before, once someone has been diagnosed as having bipolar disorder it's a pretty sure bet that he will need to be maintained on medication for the rest of his life. Some practitioners, though relatively few, will treat *some* bipolar patients by medicating individual episodes of illness. The problem with this approach, though, is that it's not always easy to bring mood episodes under control. Therefore, prevention really is the best way to deal with the disorder.

I should point out that with appropriate attention to lifestyle modifications and stress management (see Chapter 7) it's possible for some people to get to the point where they can be maintained on

Be Consistent with Treatment Appointments

It's not just medication that your partner may view as unnecessary when feeling well. Some people tend to miss therapy sessions or put off the next follow-up medication visit ("I'm doing so well I don't need to see the doctor right now."). It's important that your partner keep treatment appointments *as scheduled* and not use them just for times of crisis. Your partner's doctors also need to see your mate during periods of mood stability to form an accurate picture of the course of his or her illness. If your loved one appears in the doctor's office *only* during mood episodes, the physician, or therapist, will have an incomplete understanding of the way your partner's illness has been progressing, which, in turn, could adversely affect the doctor's ability to treat your mate. Also, many psychosocial treatments for bipolar disorder—particularly those that are skills oriented (see Chapter 4)—work best when the new skills are taught during periods of relative mood stability, so it's necessary for your partner to attend sessions at these times.

lower doses of medication than they needed at one time. Actually, I am an example of someone who has been able to do this. By working hard, along with my husband, to develop a lifestyle that promotes mood stability, I now need very low doses of medicine to be okay (although, if I were under increased stress I wouldn't hesitate, with my doctor's approval, to increase my medication either as a preventive measure or as needed). Again, however, this determination should be made only in consultation with one's doctor, not on one's own or on the advice of a spouse.

"It's Not Working"

It's easy to understand why lack of efficacy leads people to discontinue their medication. Since virtually all psychiatric medications have the potential to cause troubling side effects, it really doesn't make sense for your partner to keep taking a drug if he's not experiencing symptom relief. If your partner is getting no positive effects from medication, she needs to clearly convey to the doctor that she wants to go off it. If the doctor agrees that your partner is getting no benefit from the medication, he may want to try increasing the dosage if he suspects it's not the type of medication that is the problem but how much of it your partner is receiving. But if he determines that, in fact, this medication is not right for your mate, it's important for the doctor to be in charge of how your partner goes about stopping the medication. Although some drugs can be stopped abruptly without problems, others need to be reduced slowly—patients need to be "weaned" off them.

As I discussed in Chapter 2, although they are *significantly* better, some people don't fully—that is, 100%—recover from their mood episodes. (Others just need the addition of another medication—see the sidebar on page 154—in order to return to their pre-illness selves.) In a case like this your partner may believe a medication isn't working for her while everyone else can clearly see that it is. Maybe your partner's symptoms are less frequent and/or less severe and she is less impaired than without this medication but she continues to have some symptoms and/or signs of decreased functioning.

What can you do when your partner's perception differs from what you and the doctors can see? Daily mood charting, explained in

Chapter 7, can point out patterns and trends toward improvement that your partner might otherwise overlook. It also can be helpful for you to point out the improvements you've observed in your partner's mood state: "Honey, you used to be depressed every day all day; now it's happening only 1 or 2 days a week and you're able to get out of it in a few hours." Or draw your partner's attention to improvements in specific bothersome symptoms: "You couldn't sleep at all when you were manic—

Criteria for Improvement
- Less severe symptoms
- Less frequent symptoms
- Less functional impairment

now you're sleeping at least 4 to 6 hours a night" or "You couldn't sit still and watch a half-hour sitcom on television. Now you can." If your partner can now do things that he or she couldn't do during a full-blown mood episode, such as working full-time, doing chores, or pursuing his or her hobbies, note that too: "When you were depressed, you were late to work almost every day; now you're always on time" or "You're working on your scrapbooking—when you were ill, you didn't do that."

As I'll discuss in Chapter 7, it's also not unusual for people who've had mood episodes to misinterpret normal variations in mood as evidence of a mood problem. Because they've suffered so much from past mood episodes, people can become hyperalert and overreact to insignificant daily fluctuations in mood. In addition to possibly causing

Improved but Not Well

When a person is significantly improved but continues to show signs or symptoms of mood disorder, the physician often will add another medication to the patient's drug regimen rather than discontinuing the one the individual already is on. If the current drug has produced a clinically meaningful change in your partner's condition, an additional drug will often handle the residual symptoms and return your partner to a normal mood and the pre-illness level of functioning. This is one of the reasons why many bipolar people are maintained on more than one medication.

your mate to incorrectly assess the effectiveness of his medication, this type of overanxious reaction can actually bring on a mood problem, so that the person's initially unfounded concern ends up becoming a self-fulfilling prophecy.

"I Forget to Take It"

Riley hasn't stopped her medication, but she doesn't take it on a regular basis. She takes it when she remembers to, skipping a few days at a time, and is often late picking up her refills. Even though her psychiatrist has told her she needs to take her medication religiously, she pooh-poohs his advice. "It's a hassle to remember to take it every day," she says.

"Forgetting" to take one's medication can be a form of denying, or at least minimizing, the seriousness of bipolar illness. To complicate matters, most of the medications used to treat bipolar disorder remain in one's system for many days or even weeks, so skipping doses doesn't produce immediate negative effects. As a result, people can do okay for a while without their medications, which they then interpret as further proof that they don't need them. Eventually, though, missed medication will take its toll, increasing the likelihood of future mood episodes.

If your mate really has a problem remembering to take medicine—that is, it's not a reflection of denial or due to some other reason—a number of procedures can help:

- Use a watch that has a programmable alarm as a reminder that it's time to take the medication.
- Use a large pillbox that's segmented for the different days of the week.
- Keep a chart or calendar in a highly visible place, like on the refrigerator or on the bathroom mirror, and check off when a dose of medication has been taken.
- Keep medication in a highly visible place, like on the nightstand in the bedroom or on the kitchen counter, so that it's less likely to be overlooked.
- Pair the taking of medication with another daily activity, like

eating breakfast or brushing teeth, or with a certain time of the day (such as bedtime).

The "fixes" for forgetting one's medications, as you can see, are not that complicated. It can be far more difficult, however, to know when and how to broach the subject of lack of medication compliance with your spouse.

If your loved one is inconsistent in taking medication, do you just go out and buy a watch with an alarm or a pill container for him? Will your spouse get angry that you are "taking over," or will he be pleased that you've shown concern for his health? The answer to these questions depends to a large extent on the reason for the lack of adherence. If it truly is because of forgetting to take the medication, offering suggestions like the ones I've just outlined probably will be greeted with appreciation, or at least not with anger. However, if your significant other doesn't like the idea of taking medication, can't tolerate the side effects, or doesn't want to give up the manic highs, then even bringing up the subject of medication consistency is likely to be met with bristling or worse. In any of these cases, go ahead and use the strategies I've outlined in the relevant section of this chapter.

I can tell you, though, that asking your mate night after night or morning after morning whether she is taking her medication is very annoying and can make your partner feel like a child whose misbehavior you're trying to prevent. You are much better off empowering your partner with concrete solutions that can help your loved one establish the habit of regularly taking medication, again assuming that really is your mate's goal.

I virtually never forget my psychiatric medication, which I take at bedtime, but, on the other hand, I often do skip my morning vitamins. Forgetting to take my vitamins probably is occurring for one of two possible reasons—either I don't regard them as important to my health (at least not as much as I do my psychiatric drugs) or the morning isn't the best time for me to take them. If the latter is the case, it would make sense for me to switch the time I take my vitamins to the evening, the same time I take my bipolar medication. If the former is the case, than I need to develop a better appreciation for the role that vitamins play in my life, perhaps by further educating myself on the subject.

"I Can't Stand the Side Effects"

Lana has definitely been more even-keeled since taking the medications the psychiatrist prescribed. She no longer has the horrible depressions where she lies in bed with the covers over her head telling her husband, Carl, she wants to die. She also doesn't have the angry, irritable periods anymore when she picks fights with just about anybody but most of all with him.

Although she's grateful her mood is so stable, to be honest Lana misses certain aspects of her "old self." Usually a real go-getter, she's now complacent and apathetic much of the time, content doing nothing or just going along with whatever Carl suggests. Her typically sharp mind has been affected too—she's often unable to recall words and events and takes longer to catch on to things than she used to.

As you know from Chapter 4, many of the medications used for bipolar disorder have unpleasant side effects. In fact, **besides lack of efficacy, side effects are the number one reason people discontinue their medication.**

Your partner should know that many side effects of psychiatric medications go away as treatment progresses. If they persist, though, as in Lana's case, physicians will sometimes reduce the dose in an attempt to eliminate or at least lessen their severity while maintaining a therapeutic level of the drug (this is also the approach taken if an individual is overmedicated—see the sidebar on page 159). An alternative is for the doctor to prescribe another medication that gets rid of the side effect (for example, using beta-blockers to control fine motor tremors of the hands for patients on lithium). Finally, if all else fails, the physician often will consider switching to another medication that generally does not have the same side effect.

In some cases, though, the medication that's needed to keep bipolar symptoms under wraps has a significant side effect that can't be avoided.

Bradley found that he couldn't compose music—a pastime he was passionate about—when maintained on a mood stabilizer. But without the medication he was subject to "black manias" (psychotic manias with frightening hallucinations and delusions), and he was absolutely panic-stricken at the thought of their returning. Bradley had to come to terms with the limitations of having bipolar illness or, more exactly, the limitations he experienced as a result of its treatment. His wife, Shelly, helped him deal with—essentially grieve for—the loss of his ability to write music by talking with him about it and letting him express what he was experiencing:

Bradley: I feel so lost without writing music. It was such an important part of my identity.

Shelly: I know. You really put so much of yourself into it.

Bradley: I don't know how I can accept this. But, on the other hand, I can't handle this illness. I need the medication.

Shelly: Most illnesses have some sort of restrictions associated with them. Look at people who are in accidents and end up in wheelchairs, or people who have heart disease and have to modify their diets and their activity levels.

Bradley: I know, I never really thought about it before. I guess I just have to focus on what I can do with bipolar disorder, not what I no longer can do.

Shelly: I think you're right. Focus on what you can do.

On this occasion Bradley's wife served as an effective sounding board, but it's not always easy to listen and reflect back the way Shelly did. If your mate has a therapist, it may be better to let this person help your partner through the process of grieving for the loss of his "old self" and accepting the new one.

Sometimes people just need to find a better way to handle the negative effects of medication that has such a positive effect on their lives. Significant others often are in a position to help their partners better tolerate the side effects that accompany their medications, as Susan did with her husband, Chad:

Chad: Susan, I'm not as sharp as I used to be. This medication is slowing my thinking and affecting my memory.

Susan: Sweetie, all medications have side effects. You just have to get used to them.

Chad: I'm not going to get used to being *stupid*!

Susan: You're not stupid. And, honestly, you're now much more like the rest of us. You were *too* sharp before—you

---

Is Your Partner Overmedicated?

The presence of any of the following should alert you to the possibility that your partner may be overmedicated:

- Slurred speech
- Trouble walking
- Extreme lethargy
- Daytime sedation (sleepy, taking naps)
- Apathy
- Confusion

---

couldn't wait for people to finish what they were saying because you felt an urgency to interject what you wanted to say. And you had zero tolerance for people you felt weren't as smart as you.

Chad: But what about my work? How can I do my job like this?

Susan: My guess is you'll do an even better job. Now that you're more level you'll be more consistent at work. You probably won't have the on-and-off periods you had before.

Susan helped Chad gain some perspective on the side effects he was experiencing. Not only were they not as disabling as he thought, but they actually might in some ways be advantageous. You may be able to find a way to do the same with your partner.

As you know from Chapter 4, a lot of the medications used for mood stabilization (lithium, anticonvulsants, atypical antipsychotics) have weight gain as a side effect. Let's see how Donald dealt with Carol on this subject:

Carol: I must have put on 10 pounds since I started taking this medication!

Donald: Really, I haven't noticed it, but if you say so I believe you.

Carol: You can't see that I'm fat?

Donald: You always look great to me. And to tell you the truth, I wouldn't care what you weighed. I just want you to have some peace, to be rid of the mood swings.

Carol: Well, I don't want to trade one problem for another! So I won't be depressed from the bipolar disorder, but I'll be depressed from my clothes not fitting!

Donald: You know, I could stand to lose some weight. Why don't we join that new gym that opened down the road? We could work out together. That would help both of us to control our weight.

Donald initially tried to help Carol accept the extra weight she had put on by showing her how the benefits of the medication outweighed the disadvantages. When that didn't work, he came up with a potential solution to the problem—exercising—and to make the solution even more appealing to his wife he proposed that they go to the gym together as a couple.

I unfortunately am one of those people who have had weight gain as a consequence of the medications they take. And believe me, if there were any other way to have mood stability that didn't involve gaining weight I would be immediately on board for it. I've been thin virtually all of my adult life (not that I'm that big now, just bigger than before) and taken pride in my figure. So it really felt like a loss to me to have to give up the shape I liked for a less desirable one. In fact, I felt pretty sorry for myself, thinking, "Not only do I have to have bipolar disorder, but the treatment I need for it is taking away something that's important to me!"

As Donald helped Carol, my husband has helped me deal with this side effect. He frequently compliments me on my appearance, and it certainly is good to hear. Also, as the cook in our family he has made a considerable effort to come up with low-calorie meals. And when we make plans to go out for dinner, he gives thought to which restaurants would make it easiest for me to stay on my diet, such as places that have fish, salads, and the like.

I also find that when I look in the mirror and am not so pleased with what I see, it helps to say to myself, "I'd rather be one size larger and not have mood episodes." You might consider saying something like this to your spouse as well.

"I Miss My Up Periods"

Some people regard their manias and hypomanias as positive. Because they enjoy or believe they benefit from them, they're reluctant to take medication that diminishes these states.

My hypomanias made me feel creative, energized, optimistic, and confident. Who wouldn't want to feel like that? Not only did it feel good, but other people (including my husband) loved to be around me when I was this way. And since I was able to focus well during these times, my work tended to flourish too.

The problem, though, was that horrendous downs always followed my ups, so in the end the hypomanic periods weren't worth it. But to be honest with you, it did take me a number of years before I truly realized that I had to let go of the highs in order to avoid the lows.

It's not just hypomanic people who can enjoy their elevated states. Individuals with bipolar I disorder who have euphoric, nonpsychotic manias also may find them pleasurable. They focus on their feelings of elation and ignore the problematic behaviors that go along with it.

When Ling came to see me, he told me that like clockwork each winter he would get severely depressed, but that each summer he would have a manic episode. He went on to say that he took his medications religiously in the winter because the depressions were so unbearable, but stopped them in the summers because he loved his manic periods. One serious problem with this routine was that he was heavily "self-medicating" his manic raciness with alcohol and frequently driving under the influence.

Dale and Charlotte showed up together for Dale's first visit. Dale was clearly "up"—effusive, bubbly, funny, and overall generally engaging. Charlotte complained that Dale would not take a mood stabilizer because he felt that the way he currently was reflected his true self. In other words, he didn't consider the highs a problem. However, on speaking further with the couple, and also having a session with Charlotte alone, it became clear that Dale's manias had serious consequences: compulsive gambling, physical fights with strangers (and getting in trouble with the law), and spending large sums of money (that they couldn't afford) on lavish gifts for his wife.

When dealing with someone who is reluctant to let go of the highs, there really are only two lines of reasoning you can use to convince the individual that he would be better off taking medication to stabilize his mood. The first is the negative consequences that stem from manic or hypomanic behavior. The second is the depression that, for most people, follows.

The checklist on the next page lists problematic situations that can be caused by manic and hypomanic moods. Take a look at the list and check off any that have ever applied to your partner. Once you are aware of the specific problems that your significant other's highs have caused, you can use this information to help your mate see the other, not so wonderful, side of the ups. As an example, let's take a look at how Beth handled this with her husband, Norman.

Beth: Norman, you need to go back on the mood stabilizer the doctor prescribed for you.

Norman: I don't know what you're talking about. I feel great. Never better.

Beth: You might feel great, but you're not acting great. You're causing a lot of trouble for this family. It's not fair to the rest of us, or you either, for that matter.

Norman: What's your problem? You should be happy that I'm finally feeling good, not getting on my case!

Beth: Look at the facts, Norman. When you were taking your medication, you hardly ever drank, maybe an occasional glass of wine. Now you're drinking half a fifth of vodka every night.

Norman: So I like to drink. So what?

Beth: And when you drink, you get nasty. You can't tolerate the noise the kids make, and you scream at them. They're becoming frightened of you.

Norman: Oh.

Beth: And what about the days you've missed from work because you're hung over? How long do you think your boss is going to let that go by?

Negative Consequences
of Manic/Hypomanic Moods

____ Excessive alcohol or illicit drug use

____ Driving under the influence

____ Shoplifting

____ Yelling at people

____ Physical fights

____ Paranoid behavior

____ Excessive gambling

____ Excessive spending

____ Trouble with the law

____ Obsessive sexual behavior (for example, consumed with visiting strip clubs, watching pornography, etc.)

____ Sexual infidelity

____ Risky business ventures or financial investments

____ Trouble with daily functioning (performance at work, taking care of children, paying bills or meeting other responsibilities, etc.)

____ Alienating people (friends, relatives, acquaintances) with inappropriate behavior

____ Car accidents

From *When Someone You Love Is Bipolar* by Cynthia G. Last. Copyright 2009 by Cynthia G. Last.

Norman: I don't know.

Beth: And what about our friends? You were so flirtatious with Edith the last time we went out with her and Billy that they'll probably never see us again.

Norman: I was just trying to have a good time. I didn't mean anything by it.

> *Beth:*   Listen, Norman, the good time you're having is creating
>   havoc in our lives. If you care about your family and the
>   life we have, you have to do the right thing and go back
>   on your medication.

Beth had to have this conversation with her husband several times before it finally paid off. Eventually, by Beth's repeatedly pointing out how his hypomania was causing trouble in almost all areas of their lives, Norman was forced to face what he had chosen, in his elevated mood state, to ignore.

Not everyone is as easy to convince as Norman. The allure of an elevated mood can be very strong, and the capacity of human beings for denial equally strong. Jacob had to have his driver's license suspended for a DUI before he agreed to go back on his medication. Ann almost lost her fiancé because she had an affair with another man while she was taking "a vacation" from her mood stabilizer. Patty's manic spending sprees led her and her husband to have to file for bankruptcy before Patty finally "saw the light"—that she *had to* take her medication regularly.

I hope you and your mate's doctor will be able to persuade your loved one to forgo the highs and avoid the potentially catastrophic consequences that manic moods can bring. If you can't, though, and your spouse—and you too—has to suffer negative consequences before changing her behavior, see how to get past the rubble and again look forward to the future in Chapter 10.

In this chapter I've discussed the different reasons your partner may not adhere to his or her medication regimen and what you can do—and can't do—to help your loved one become more compliant. In the next chapter I'll be talking about other things you and your mate can do to help prevent mood episodes, including mood monitoring and identifying mood triggers, making certain lifestyle modifications, and reducing stress and conflict.

Other Things You and Your Partner Can Do to Prevent Mood Episodes

Ever since his hospitalization and diagnosis of bipolar disorder, Hayden has taken his medication religiously. But although he's followed his doctor's advice on this, he has ignored warnings about other things he should be doing to prevent mood episodes. One of those things—quitting drinking—is a particular sore point between him and his wife, Ellen:

Ellen: *Hayden, you've got to stop drinking.*

Hayden: *It's bad enough that I have bipolar disorder. I shouldn't have to give up everything in my life because of this illness!*

Ellen: *But the drinking is a big problem. You get really angry and sometimes even mean when you've had a few, from Dr. Jekyll to Mr. Hyde, a lot like how you are when you're manic.*

Hayden: *I don't believe that.*

Ellen: *Ask your family, or our friends, and see what they have to say. I know your brother has commented*

> *to me many times about the personality switch you have when you're drinking.*

Hayden: *Well, you know Jeff's opinion on alcohol. Of course he's going to see a problem with my drinking.*

Ellen: *But other people have said things to me too. Like last week when we went out with Beth and Mathew. You were making a lot of sarcastic jokes, and Beth turned to me and said, "I can't believe the things Hayden says about you—how do you handle it?"*

Hayden: *I thought I was being funny.*

Ellen: *You're not funny—you're nasty—and it's frequently at my expense.*

Hayden: *You know I love you.*

Ellen: *I know, but when you drink you're not that person.*

Hayden: *I'm sorry.*

Ellen: *I don't want you to be sorry. I want you to stop drinking. And if you don't want to stop for you and your health, then stop for me and for us. Do it for our relationship.*

As you know from the preceding chapter, being consistent with medication is an absolute prerequisite to staying well. Without it your partner's chance of having another mood episode increases dramatically. But while pharmacological treatment is *necessary* for bipolar mental health, it is not by itself *sufficient*. Staying well involves attending to a number of factors that have been shown to affect mood health.

Many chronic illnesses—not only bipolar disorder—necessitate making lifestyle changes. For instance, in the case of heart disease people usually are advised to alter their diet, to exercise, and to decrease stress to promote heart health. Similarly, bipolar disorder is impacted by its own set of risk factors, and people with this illness benefit immensely from paying attention to them.

In this chapter I'll be talking about the specific things your mate can do—alone or together with you—that will affect the course of his or her illness. These measures all involve minimizing one of the factors mentioned in Chapter 2 that are associated with an increased risk of illness recurrence or, looking at it from a different perspective, maximizing those that serve a protective function. Some involve learning about and making certain lifestyle changes that promote wellness—like abstaining from alcohol, getting sufficient sleep, and having a regular daily routine of activities—while others focus on acquiring skills and using techniques that help keep stress and anxiety low, such as resolving interpersonal conflicts and avoiding (when possible) stressful life events.

Some of the preventive measures that your partner will need to take will affect you too—as well as your life together. Some will impact your daily habits and routines, such as your spouse's need to go to bed and eat meals at a regular time. Others will affect more occasional aspects of your life, like vacation plans. Still others will influence some of the important life decisions that the two of you will make, such as moving, changing jobs, or even having children (see Chapter 10 for more on this very important subject).

At times you may find your greatest contribution will be encouraging your partner to take the first step toward making a change or supporting your loved one's efforts to stick with a preventive measure that he finds unappealing. Other times you may find more is required of you, possibly involving certain sacrifices on your part. What kinds of changes you will need to make depends on a number of factors, and how active you are in helping your partner with these is, of course, ultimately up to you. But what my husband and I have found, and many of my patients and their partners have discovered too, is that with time and trial and error you eventually come up with a "collaboration," if you will, that works. As a team, my husband and I have been able to put our prevention plan successfully into effect. Stay the course and I'm sure you and your mate will be able to achieve this too.

Encourage Your Partner to Learn about Bipolar Disorder

Psychoeducation—becoming knowledgeable about bipolar disorder—is the most basic, but often overlooked, means of helping people avoid future mood episodes. I've already emphasized the importance of your learning about bipolar disorder. But it's essential for your partner to learn about the illness too. That's because understanding the nature of the illness—including what increases the risk of having additional episodes (see the sidebar below) and what serves as protection from them—equips people to make wise choices about how they live their lives. For example, knowing that sleep deprivation is strongly associated with illness recurrence can help influence your partner to make rest a priority. And knowing the kinds of stressors that are likely to trigger mood episodes can help steer your mate away from potentially problematic situations.

Learning from the Doctors

One way for your partner to learn about bipolar illness is by getting information from her own doctors. You should be aware, however, that mental health professionals vary in how comfortable they are sharing information with their patients. Generally speaking, psychologists usually are more apt to take a proactive role in educating people than psychiatrists, although this has been changing in recent years as physicians are being better trained to meet their patients' need for information.

The value of the information obtained from doctors often rests on the questions that patients themselves raise. If you accompany your partner to medication management or therapy appointments (as I encouraged you to do in Chapter 5), you can help facilitate this pro-

---

Factors That Increase the Risk of Future Mood Episodes

- Decreased sleep
- Anxiety
- Substance abuse
- Stressful life events
- Interpersonal conflict
- Disruptions in usual daily and evening routines
- Medication inconsistency

Questions for the Doctor

- "Besides medication, what currently are the most effective treatments (therapies) for bipolar disorder? Is there one (or more) that you recommend specifically for my spouse?"
- "Are there other things (besides medication; therapy) that you suggest my partner do to help keep control of his or her illness?"
- "From what you've observed, is there anything in particular that you think may be an obstacle or especially challenging for my partner?"
- "What's likely to make my partner worse? Better (other than the things we already talked about)?"

cess by asking questions of your own. Some suggestions for topics you might want to touch on are listed in the sidebar above.

Self-Help Books

There are other ways to increase one's knowledge about bipolar illness besides getting information from the doctors. As I mentioned in Chapter 3, there are a number of excellent self-help books for people who have bipolar disorder (some of which are listed in the Resources at the back of this book).

However, if your spouse is in denial about or minimizing the significance of his illness, it's unlikely that he is going to—on his own—purchase a book about his illness. In a situation like this some individuals will respond positively to their partners' taking the lead and bringing something home for them to read. Alternatively—and you have to be the judge of this, given what you know about your loved one—your mate may react with anger and then refuse even to look at the book, let alone read it. In this case I suggest *you* obtain and then read the book—and that you do so, at least some of the time, in front of your partner.

Why should you read about bipolar disorder? As I've already said, it's important that you learn about the disorder so you can help your mate. But just as important, I think it's probable that your mate will develop a curiosity about what you're reading and will look at the book, given it's in your home. If, however, she does not do this, she can still reap the benefits of what you've learned if you share information from what you've read.

Although, obviously, I don't rely on my husband for information on bipolar disorder because of the knowledge I already have in this area, I've been faced recently with another medical situation that I've been avoiding paying attention to. Now in my 50s, I have started to go through menopause, a phase of life that is accompanied by a number of not-so-pleasant changes.

Seeing that I was "sticking my head in the sand" when it came to learning about menopause, my husband took it upon himself to search the Internet for information that might be relevant to what I was experiencing. And from time to time, when I would be concerned about a particular symptom (like hot flashes, fluid retention, etc.), he would step in and share an important fact about menopause with me, not only giving me information but also providing me with the support and reassurance I needed.

The Internet

Another avenue for learning about bipolar disorder is for your partner to make use of the Internet by visiting websites devoted to the illness (again, see Resources). However, if, again, your mate does not want to put forth this effort (because of denial or for any other reason), there's certainly nothing to stop you from doing the legwork and then sharing with your loved one what you've found by passing along articles or verbalizing tidbits of information from them. (Referring again to my situation, my husband printed out several articles for me about menopause in the hope of getting me started on learning about it. Guess what? It worked.)

Anne tended to be a "night owl," often going to bed at 2:00 A.M. or even later and frequently not getting enough sleep. However, when she and her husband went together to a manic–depressive support group, one of the participants mentioned that his doctor had told him about the relationship between keeping routines—including having a set time to go to sleep—and mood stability. Once armed with this knowledge, Anne made a real effort to normalize her sleep as well as several of her other daily routines.

Interacting with Others Who Have Bipolar Disorder

Your partner can learn more about bipolar disorder by interacting with others who have the illness, either in online chat rooms or, like Anne, by attending a support or self-help group. If your loved one is interested in going to a group but hesitant to attend alone, you can offer to go along, assuming the group is open to nonbipolar participants.

Support Your Partner in Monitoring Mood and Identifying Mood Triggers

Mood monitoring can help your partner become more aware of mood fluctuations and the variables that influence them. In fact, monitoring mood and identifying factors associated with mood changes are essential components of many of the skills-oriented therapies reviewed in Chapter 4. Generally, your partner would assign and record an overall numerical score for mood for each day, using a rating scale designed for this purpose, also noting any significant events—"mood triggers"—that may be related to the mood fluctuations.

Although intended primarily as a self-help strategy, in certain circumstances the monitoring can be done by someone close to the ill person. Specifically, it may be helpful for you to handle this task if your spouse:

- Can't—because of the severity of his illness—or won't, because of denial or minimization of the illness, do it on his own.
- Tends to over- or underestimate the severity of her own mood states.
- Needs or wants your help in learning to chart moods.
- Wants external validation of his own perceptions of his mood states.

If you decide to take on monitoring, make sure your mate doesn't end up using you as an out to avoid having to take care of her own illness. Remember, your goal is *to help* your partner take better care of herself, not to take this job on yourself.

Also keep in mind that your ability to observe what's going on with your partner's moods is limited by the fact that you're observing from the outside. *Objective behaviors*—such as the things your mate does and says—that go along with different mood states may be easy to spot, but only your partner may be privy to other types of information. For example, taking an extreme case, if your partner is depressed and having suicidal thoughts but hasn't shared them with you, you're not going to be in as good a position to assess the level of severity of his depression as he is. What this means, then, is that if your partner rates his mood as more severe than you do, you should ask questions before assuming he's incorrectly evaluating his own condition. You may ask, in a situation like this, "Is there anything I don't know about that's making you rate your mood as more depressed [or manic] than I am?"

By keeping tabs on where your partner is with respect to her mood, you and your loved one—and, when indicated, the doctors—will be able to:

1. Determine whether a new treatment (medication or therapy) or recently implemented lifestyle change (such as getting regular sleep) is having the desired effect.
2. Detect the onset of a potential mood episode early on so that it can be nipped in the bud (I'll be talking about early identification and early intervention at length in Chapters 8 and 9).
3. Identify precipitants and patterns to mood fluctuations, by simultaneously keeping track of significant events (to be discussed later on in this section).

Step 1: Learn to Use the Mood Rating Scale

The very first step in monitoring mood is to become familiar with the mood scale on pages 174–175. The scale, as you can see, spans from a low of –4 (severe depression) to a high of +4 (severe mania) and is based both on the severity of current symptoms and the degree of impairment in functioning they cause. Normal mood is rated as a "0" and indicates that no signs of mania or depression are present and your partner is functioning normally in all areas (at work or school, socially and in close relationships). A score of "1" indicates that your loved one is at the "top" (+1) or "bottom" (–1) of normal; a score of "2" indicates that he is hypomanic (+2) or mildly depressed (–2); a rating of "3" means that he is moderately manic (+3) or moderately depressed (–3); and a "4" is used to denote severe mania (+4) or severe depression (–4).

Many people whose partners have just been diagnosed really don't know what the different symptoms of mania and depression typically look like. By familiarizing yourself with the mood scale, you'll have something concrete to judge your mate's moods on instead of always wondering "Is this mania? How can I be sure this is a problem? What if I jump the gun and start assuming the worst when nothing's really happening?" Or the opposite, overlooking important indicators that suggest a problem *is* beginning to rear its head.

By becoming acquainted with the mood scale, Craig learned that Stella's out-of-control rages were signs of moderate-to-severe mania that required her doctor's attention. After reading the description of mild depression, Kate realized that Andrew's "alone time" might be an indicator of a mood shift.

Your observations of your mate's behavior, including the things she says out loud, will help you formulate the mood rating for your partner at any given point in time. At first it may seem a bit complicated to choose among the different gradations of the mood scale, but after becoming more familiar with it through practice I know you'll find it pretty easy.

As a small exercise, right now, consider where your mate is in respect to his mood today, using the mood scale. Is he pretty much normal (anywhere from a –1 to a +1)? Is he mildly or moderately depressed (–2 or –3), that is, noticeably down or withdrawn, or manic (+2 or +3), that is, obviously up, agitated, or angry but still able to take care of some or all of his responsibilities? Or is he severely ill, at an extreme end of the scale, unable to function at all, quite possibly even requiring hospitalization (–4 or +4)?

Once you've determined the overall area of the scale that currently applies to your mate, you can narrow it even further. For instance, if the mood is normal, is it on the high or "up" side of normal, with your mate being cheerful and optimistic (+1)? Or on the low side of normal, a bit quiet, subdued, or lethargic (–1)? Or, possibly, neither of these but just plain "normal" (0)?

If your mate's mood falls in the mild-to-moderate portion of the scale, are the symptoms obvious to others and/or is there some reduction in functioning ("moderate"—a –3 or +3)? Or are the signs of the

Mood Rating Scale

+4 Severely manic. Ecstatic or full of rage; uncontrollable laughter or anger; may be paranoid and/or violent; nonstop talking—may "trip" over words; may make up words or is incoherent; barely sleeping or not sleeping at all; may have delusions or hallucinations (grandiose or paranoid); unable to sit still; racing thoughts or "flight of ideas" (images that race through the mind); completely unable to focus; no judgment; risk-taking behavior; public displays that lead to the attention of the police; depressive symptoms also may be present; unable to perform usual activities; hospitalization necessary.

Your partner may say: "I feel out of control," "I feel like hurting you [him, her, etc.]," "I have special powers," "_____ is out to get me," "I'm going crazy," "I need to be in a hospital," "I can't think straight," "I'm having a breakdown."

+3 Moderately manic. Elated, "high," euphoric, and/or extremely angry or irritable and anxious; suspicious or paranoid; hyperactive; inflated self-esteem; can't stop talking; needs very little sleep; highly distractible; racing thoughts; may have rage attacks when crossed or verbally abusive to others; poor judgment and risk-taking behavior; hypersexual; depressive symptoms also may be present; functioning is definitely impaired and is noticeable by others.

Your partner may say: "I'm on top of the world," "Nothing can go wrong," "Everyone's moving [talking, working, etc.] too slowly," "I hate you [him, her, etc.]," "I feel paranoid," "I'm manic," "I feel like breaking things."

+2 Hypomanic (mildly manic). Predominant mood is "up," very happy, boisterous, irritable, or angry; energetic; full of ideas and projects; increased libido; gregarious; talkative; may want to travel, spend money, gamble; requires less sleep than usual; optimistic, self-confident; may exhibit poor judgment and risk-taking behavior; may have some trouble paying attention; functioning is not really impaired and may be perceived as better than normal.

Your partner may say: "I feel terrific," "Everything is getting on my nerves," "I'm more social," "I'm feeling sexy," "Everything's going my way," "My brain is working faster than usual."

+1 Hyperthymic. Cheerful; optimistic; witty; energetic; sociable; decisive; sometimes irritable; functioning at or slightly above normal.

Your partner may say: "I feel happy," "I'm content," "Things are going well," "I'm looking forward to _____," "I wish I could feel like this all the time."

 0 Normal. No symptoms of mania or depression; functions well socially and at work

From *When Someone You Love Is Bipolar* by Cynthia G. Last. Copyright 2009 by Cynthia G. Last.

−1 Dysthymic. Low-key; somewhat pessimistic; low energy; slightly withdrawn; not very talkative; smiles infrequently; may be indecisive; may have physical complaints; functioning at or slightly below normal.

Your partner may say: "I'm tired," "I don't have anything to say," "I'm having trouble making up my mind," "I don't have much to look forward to."

−2 Mildly depressed. Mildly depressed mood—feels sad, "down in the dumps," bored, or irritable; less self-confident; less social than usual; less energetic; some loss of interest in usual activities; reduced ability to experience pleasure; negative or pessimistic; although may feel not performing at usual level, functioning appears to others to be normal.

Your partner may say: "I feel down [sad, blue, 'down in the dumps,' unhappy]," "I feel bored all the time," "I'm irritable," "I don't feel like talking," "Thing's aren't going my way," "Nothing ever works out for me," "I'm not working as well as usual," "I'm not sleeping as well as usual," "I feel bad about myself."

−3 Moderately depressed. Moderately depressed mood—feeling very sad; loss of interest or pleasure in some activities; feeling slowed down and lethargic; withdrawn; disturbed patterns of eating and sleeping; reduced libido; hopelessness; difficulty concentrating or making decisions; suicidal thoughts may be present; functioning is impaired (arriving at work late; not performing at usual level in ordinary responsibilities; some decline in self-care) and is noticeable by close friends and relatives.

Your partner may say: "I must have done something wrong," "Nothing will ever work out for me," "I'm bad," "I wish I was dead," "I can't think straight," "I feel slowed down," "Time seems to be going slowly," "Food doesn't taste the same."

−4 Severely depressed. Profoundly sad or numb; completely withdrawn; loss of interest in all activities; inability to experience pleasure; no energy; no appetite; severely disturbed sleep (sleeping all the time or inability to sleep); feels guilty or worthless, hopeless; suicidal; may have delusions and/or hallucinations (for example, is being punished by God); functioning is markedly impaired—can't work or perform usual activities, doesn't take care of basic elements of self-care (like grooming, washing clothes); voluntary or involuntary (to prevent harm to self) hospitalization may be necessary.

Your partner may say: "I don't feel anything," "I can't eat," "I can't sleep," "I can't stop crying," "I'm worthless," "I'm being punished," "I want to die," "I can't think," "I need to go to a hospital," "I feel like I'm in a tunnel," "I feel like there's a black cloud (black veil) over my head."

illness hard to notice (obvious only to you and those really close to your partner), with no significant loss of functioning ("mild"—a –2 or +2)?

Step 2: Work on Identifying Mood Triggers

The second step in the process of monitoring mood involves becoming more aware of events and situations that may be associated with mood swings. To begin to get a handle on this, you, your mate, or the two of you (together or separately) should fill out the mood trigger inventory on page 177. The inventory lists many different environmental and bio-logical/physiological circumstances that frequently are associated with mood fluctuations. Some of the items included in the list are major life events—like having a baby or moving to a new residence—while others are more common but also potentially mood triggering—like the tim-ing of a woman's menstrual cycle, conflicts with others, and reduced sleep (some of these are discussed at length later on in this chapter).

The benefit to having your input on the inventory (by filling it out together with or independently from your mate) is that you may be aware of associations that aren't apparent to your loved one. For instance, in the example that appeared at the very beginning of this chapter, Ellen was able to identify a relationship between alcohol and an angry, nasty maniclike mood in her husband, Hayden.

In talking about identifying potential causes of mood fluctuations, I should mention that sometimes people can get into a "chicken and egg" dilemma when it comes to looking at the relationship between mood ratings and so-called "triggers." That is, they may be so closely related in time that it can be difficult to know *which came first*—the mood fluctuation *or* the event. For example, when people are becoming hypomanic, they may get irritable, which in turn can lead to conflicts with people around them. However, conflicts with other people—because of the anxiety they produce—also *can precipitate* the develop-ment of hypomania. To complicate the matter even further, using the same example, conflicts that emerge as a result of being hypomanic can exacerbate and escalate a mild mood problem into a more severe one so that they really can be thought of *as both* a consequence—of an already existing hypomanic episode—and a precipitant, of a more severe state of illness.

Another example is reduced sleep. As I'll discuss in more depth

Mood Triggers

Place a check next to all events or circumstances that you think have been associated with significant mood fluctuations or precipitated mood episodes in the past.

____ Marital or relationship conflict

____ Minor physical illness, like a cold, back pain, etc.

____ Missing a meal

____ Stress at work

____ Making a large purchase

____ Losing a job

____ Jet lag

____ Car accident

____ Death or serious physical illness in the family

____ Getting a pet

____ Pregnancy

____ Postpartum period

____ Vacations

____ Moving

____ Menopause

____ Anxiety or panic attacks

____ Certain medications—*specify*: _____

____ Menstrual cycle

____ Getting less sleep than usual

____ Going to sleep later than usual

____ Excessive social stimulation

____ A particular season of the year—*specify*: _____

____ Too few social interactions

____ Direct exposure to sunlight

____ Lack of sunlight

____ Alcohol or illicit drugs

____ Sleeping in

____ Lack of exercise or physical activity

____ Gambling, stock market "day trading," or other risk-taking activities

____ Other—*specify:* _____

____ Other—*specify:* _____

____ Other—*specify:* _____

From *When Someone You Love Is Bipolar* by Cynthia G. Last. Copyright 2009 by Cynthia G. Last.

later in this chapter, a decrease in sleep has been well documented to often precipitate mood episodes but also is frequently *a consequence* of abnormal mood states. And again, adding more complexity to the situation, the disturbed sleep patterns that emerge during mood episodes can then further worsen and/or prolong an existing mood problem.

Even though it may be hard to ascertain the direction of the relationship in specific instances, when you begin to actually monitor and look at many occurrences over weeks or months, the nature of the association should become clear. If it doesn't, though, it probably is because of the scenario I just outlined—that is, the identified trigger is functioning as both a cause and a consequence.

Step 3: Start Charting with the Mood Monitoring Form

Once you're sufficiently familiar with the mood rating scale and you've begun to identify possible mood triggers, you can start the process of daily monitoring. While it's certainly fine to keep this information in your head, only to be shared with your mate (or your mate's doctors) in the event of a significant fluctuation (either up or down the scale), you may find it easier instead to actually jot down scores using a form designated for this purpose, like the one on page 179. (If you don't want to use a form, it's also possible to keep track of mood more informally by recording daily ratings in a date book or on a calendar, in a notebook or journal, or using some other device—like a computer—that's convenient.) However, *please do not physically chart in writing your mate's mood without checking first that this is okay with your partner.* If you don't and your partner discovers what you've been doing, he may feel spied on or that you've been "keeping a secret." The only exception to this would be if your mate is showing psychotic features, in which case sharing what you want to do might be misconstrued—because of your partner's trouble with perceiving reality—as harmful rather than helpful.

If you choose to use the mood chart, give your partner an *overall* rating for her mood for each day of the week. For best accuracy, assign the mood rating at the end of the day rather than waiting till the next morning or the end of the week. Then note in the "possible triggers" column for the day any stressful or other potentially significant events or life circumstances that you think might have had or possibly will have mood ramifications. These may include situations that are listed

---

Mood Monitoring Form

	Mood rating (−4 to +4)	Possible triggers
Monday	_____	_____
Tuesday	_____	_____
Wednesday	_____	_____
Thursday	_____	_____
Friday	_____	_____
Saturday	_____	_____
Sunday	_____	_____

From *When Someone You Love Is Bipolar* by Cynthia G. Last. Copyright 2009 by Cynthia G. Last.

---

in the mood trigger inventory or any other events that you think are relevant.

As I said earlier, monitoring mood along with trigger situations gives your partner and/or you the opportunity to *identify precipitants* of and *see patterns* in mood fluctuations, especially when examining recordings made over some time. This is important because uncovering mood triggers can put you and your partner in a position to avoid them if they are potentially avoidable. Even in the event that a trigger is unavoidable, its impact may be able to be minimized by planning ahead. For example, the doctor may adjust your loved one's medication

---

By knowing the specific situations and circumstances that cause mood fluctuations, your mate can ...

- *Avoid certain potential triggers of mood problems,* limiting alcohol, eating meals regularly, getting sufficient sleep.
- *Plan preventively for, and minimize the effects of, unavoidable mood triggers*—like seasonal mood episodes, premenstrual mood swings, jet lag.

---

in anticipation of a situation that has proved difficult for your mate in the past. Also, your mate may be able to eliminate *other* stressors—avoidable ones—during the same time period, thereby decreasing his overall level of stress.

Does Your Partner Misinterpret and Overreact to Normal Mood Fluctuations?

John is petrified of having another manic episode. He tells me that during the past week he has been feeling pretty good—upbeat, confident, and productive—but he's concerned about what this might mean. With a worried look on his face, he asks me, "Is this normal, or am I becoming manic again?" After getting more information from him, I reassure him that his "feeling good" is well within the realm of normal. John is visibly relieved.

Many people who have had full-blown mood episodes are terrified of having recurrences. Suffering through the intense emotional pain of a depressive episode or living through frightening psychotic manifestations, destructive behaviors, and the heartbreaking consequences of a manic one, they, quite understandably, will do anything to stave off another occurrence.

Unfortunately, some bipolar people become *over*vigilant for potential signs of trouble and misinterpret normal, mild variations in mood as indications of a problem. Please don't get me wrong: there is no question that it's very important to be aware of the early manifestations of a mood episode in order to nip a potential problem in the bud. However, it's also important not to become crippled by the illness so that mild, inconsequential daily fluctuations in mood are misinterpreted as a cause for alarm.

By making your partner very vigilant to mood fluctuations, mood monitoring can, in some cases, foster overconcern. That's why when using the technique I caution that both you and your mate try very hard **not to overinterpret and overreact to normal, mild variations in mood or brief periods of mildly elevated or depressed mood.** Overinterpreting and overreacting lead to anxiety, which is known to trigger mood episodes, which can create a self-fulfilling prophecy.

So how *do* you distinguish between normal variations in mood and fluctuations that suggest a budding problem? Several benchmarks can help:

- *What is the magnitude of the mood change?* A mood change of –1 or +1 is probably not significant, while a mood change greater than this may be (the greater the magnitude of the mood change, the greater the cause for concern).
- *How long has it been going on?* A minor mood shift over a brief period of time (like a couple of days) is typically of less concern than one that's gone on for some time (2 weeks or more).
- *Are "early warning signs" present?* As I discuss in Chapters 8 and 9, if one or more of your mate's characteristic early warning signs of depression or mania are present (in addition to the mood change), you have greater cause for concern (the higher the number of symptoms present, the greater the concern).

Over the last couple of days Kenneth has felt somewhat down. When he tells his wife he's scared that it could be the start of another depression, Patrice replies, "Everyone has days like this. It doesn't necessarily mean you're getting depressed." She also points out that her husband isn't showing any of his early warning symptoms of depression—trouble sleeping, giving up activities he enjoys, difficulty concentrating— further proof that what he is experiencing isn't a recurrence.

Patrice has reassured and normalized what Kenneth was going through and, in doing so, reduced his fear that he was on the road to another depressive episode. If your loved one tends to make more of minor or brief mood fluctuations than he should, you too can help by putting things into perspective, much the way Patrice did for her husband.

Encourage Your Partner to Get Sufficient Sleep

I can't underscore enough how important it is that your partner get enough sleep. As you know from Chapter 2, research shows that decreased sleep can precipitate the development of a mood episode. Also, as a symptom of an ongoing manic or depressive episode, it can increase the severity and length of an existing mood problem.

I know about the significance of sleep in bipolar illness not just from the research that's been conducted in this area. In my practice I've seen scores of people who show the same pattern—decreased sleep for one or more days followed by an elevation or dip in mood. And I've found that this relationship exists for me too—reduced sleep making me irritable and susceptible to hypomania—so that I go to great lengths to ensure that I regularly get sufficient sleep.

Making sleep a priority can involve some planning ahead. For example, I do my best to arrange social plans on weekend nights at times that won't interfere with my usual bedtime. If the scheduling of the activity is outside my control—like going to a party at someone else's home—this can involve leaving somewhat earlier than I might (under other circumstances) want to. In a case like this I have my husband—my personal cheerleader—to help motivate me to "do the right thing."

Another thing I pay attention to is the level of stimulation that my evening activities provide. For instance, in choosing a movie to watch at night that will end near my bedtime, I usually select one that isn't overchallenging intellectually or emotionally, perhaps picking a comedy or light drama instead. My husband, who is an avid movie fan, understands that "heavy" films have to be reserved for earlier in the evening or during the day—so that my mind has sufficient time to unwind before I try to go to sleep.

Might you find that making your mate's bedtime a priority is somewhat restrictive? Possibly. Even though you may usually be very supportive, it would be understandable for you to become annoyed at times at having to curtail your evening plans so that your spouse can get to sleep at her usual bedtime. But if you consider the alternative—mood instability—I think you'll agree that it's a rather small sacrifice to make.

Even with the best of intentions and plans, it's often difficult for bipolar individuals to fall asleep, particularly at times that most people would consider "normal." Many bipolar people seem to have their sleep–wake cycles somewhat reversed, so that they are at peak energy levels at night and are then ready for sleep in the morning hours—for example, at 3:00 or 4:00 A.M. Besides sleep-inducing medication, which may be prescribed for this problem, following good "sleep hygiene" (see the sidebar on the facing page) can help a lot.

Getting to Sleep

Your partner *should* ...

- Have a *regular bedtime* and a *regular wake time.*
- Engage in *relaxing activities* before going to bed, such as taking a hot bath, listening to calming music, using relaxation techniques (see the Resources for sources of more information on these methods).
- Make sure the sleep environment is *comfortable* (mattress isn't too hard or too soft; bedroom temperature is not too low or too high).
- Consider *natural remedies,* like chamomile tea or milk (it's high in the amino acid tryptophan—a sleep-including substance), or, with your doctor's approval, supplements (such as passionflower, valerian root, melatonin) that have sleep-inducing properties.

Your partner should *not* ...

- Engage in *stimulating activities* just before bedtime, like exercising, finishing up work that hasn't been completed during the day, watching a thought-provoking or scary movie.
- *Eat a heavy meal* close to bedtime.
- Take in *caffeinated products* late in the day or during the evening.
- Take *naps* during the day.
- Use the *bedroom for other activities,* like finishing up work, watching television.
- Bring *worries* into the bedroom (see page 184 for how to combat this problem).
- *Stay in bed for more than 20 minutes* if unable to fall asleep, but rather get up and engage in a quiet, relaxing activity, like reading.

Is Anxiety Keeping Your Partner Awake?

Some people have trouble falling asleep because of anxiety. In fact, anxiety itself is a well-documented trigger for mood episodes, at least in part because it interferes with getting sufficient rest (anxiety → decreased sleep → mood episode). Although anxiety is most likely to trigger hypomanic and manic moods, it also can set off depression.

(Given the prominent role it can play, learning to keep anxiety down is a central feature of certain psychosocial treatments for bipolar disorder, such as cognitive–behavioral therapy; see Chapter 4).

Anxiety has three main components: physiological, cognitive, and behavioral. The physiological component refers to bodily manifestations of anxiety, such as increased heart rate, increased blood pressure, muscle tension, and sweating. The cognitive component includes worries and catastrophic thoughts, such as "What if … ?" thoughts. The behavioral component includes "nervous habits" (nail biting, hair twirling, cracking one's knuckles, etc.) and also escape and avoidance behaviors. When people have trouble sleeping, it's often related to physiological and/or cognitive manifestations of anxiety.

If your mate feels physically keyed up at the end of the day and can't relax, he may benefit from relaxation exercises. Two popular ones frequently used by psychologists with their patients include *diaphragmatic breathing* and *deep muscle relaxation.* Diaphragmatic breathing concentrates on changing breathing patterns, while deep muscle relaxation involves tightening and then relaxing different muscles in the body. (See the Resources for sources of additional information.)

If your mate can't get to sleep because of worries that go round and round in her head, she may benefit from *scheduling worry time* into the day. (This technique also helps people who don't have trouble sleeping but suffer from excessive worrying throughout the day). Basically, the technique entails setting aside a specified period of time—usually 30 minutes or more—at a certain time of day for engaging in worrying. The worrying should be done in a quiet location, but not in the bedroom, and it never should be conducted at bedtime. People often find it helpful to conduct their worrying time in the early evening—after experiencing the trials and tribulations of the day but far enough from bedtime so as not to interfere with sleep. If your partner feels it would be helpful, and you are agreeable, you can help your mate during the worry period by serving as a sounding board (I do this with my husband, and it really helps).

Some individuals find it useful to write out their worries on paper during the worry time because they say it helps to get the thoughts "out of their heads." Writing things out also can be useful for worries that revolve around problems that need to be solved or decisions that need to be made.

Worry periods will give your mate designated times to engage in worrying so that the bed and bedtime no longer need to be used for this purpose. But if upsetting thoughts still enter your partner's head when he is trying to get to sleep, your mate needs to dismiss the worry by silently saying to himself that he will worry about whatever the concern is during the worry time that's scheduled into the next day. At first this will be difficult, but with practice it gets progressively easier, and in time, with continued use, it will become virtually automatic.

Have a Family Routine

Our routines and rituals help to anchor our lives by providing structure and predictability. Changes or disruptions in routine—including those that affect the sleep–wake cycle as well as other evening and day-time rituals and regularly scheduled events—can have a major impact on the development of mood episodes. As you learned in Chapter 4, an understanding of this relationship in part has formed the basis of interpersonal and social rhythm therapy, a treatment that can help prevent bipolar episodes.

Here are a few suggestions that your partner can use to establish good routines:

- Have a consistent time to *wake up in the morning and go to sleep at night* (see the sidebar on page 183 for tips on how to get to sleep if this is a problem for your partner), if possible the same times on weekends as on weekdays.
- Have a regular time for *going to and leaving work* or other daily obligations (volunteer work, school, home, or child care).
- Keep *mealtimes* consistent, for example, dinner at 6:30 P.M. every night.
- Have set times for *social contact*—telephone calls, face-to-face interactions (like dinner out with another couple every Saturday night; playing bridge every Thursday night; etc.).
- Have *other activities* that are regularly scheduled (like certain television shows that the family watches on particular nights; attending church on Sunday morning; a time each day to go to the gym or to work out at home).

I realize that this prescription may sound somewhat rigid. But if you really think about it, it's pretty close to the way most adults and their families live their lives. Having a regular time for doing things—like going to work (or school), eating dinner, going to sleep—is the rule rather than the exception, at least among people in this country.

However, it's also important not to be so fixed on a schedule that there's no room for any deviation. For example, if dinner normally is eaten at 6:30 P.M. on weekdays and you and your significant other plan to go out for a romantic dinner on Saturday night, making a reservation for 7:30 P.M. should not cause a problem. On the other hand, having dinner at 9:30 P.M. might be a problem, not only because of the much later mealtime but also because eating so late could end up affecting the time your partner goes to bed as well as the ability to fall asleep (see the sidebar on page 183).

It may be hard to see a change in routine as potentially detrimental to mood, especially when you view a particular change as "positive." For example, my husband and I recently had good friends of ours from out of state come for a long weekend (3 nights, 4 days). Understandably, our normal weekend routine was changed with houseguests around (different activities; different times for meals, sleep, etc.). But in addition to this was another deviation from our normal routine, one that I think most spouses of bipolar people wouldn't be aware could cause a problem—that is, the amount of "social stimulation" that comes from being with a group of people 24/7. As I might have predicted, knowing what I know about bipolar illness, all of these changes (particularly, I believe, the frequency and intensity of the social contact) resulted in my having significant trouble falling asleep. And decreased sleep can trigger a mood episode.

Fortunately, I didn't become hypomanic, which is my predisposition in the face of sleep deprivation. But I have to say that my mood for the week following their visit wasn't as stable as it usually is (some days hyperthymic or +1 on the mood scale, other days dysthymic or –1 on the scale). Let me be quick to say that this is not a reflection of how I feel about these friends or the enjoyment I got from their visit. It's just that any significant alteration in routine, such as this one, carries with it a risk of destabilization.

Changes in routine can also make vacations difficult for people who have bipolar disorder (in addition to the effect of jet lag on one's biological clock). That's why when I take a vacation I make an effort to develop "a vacation routine," certain things that I do at certain times pretty much every day while I'm away. And when my husband and I go about selecting a vacation for ourselves, we pay attention to how easy (or difficult) it will be to formulate a routine for me on the trip. For instance, a vacation that involves staying at a different location every night or two would be much more stressful for me than spending a whole week (or more) in one location. In fact, living in South Florida and being so close to the ports for many cruise lines, I find that cruising is an excellent choice for a vacation for me because it allows me to formulate a routine on the ship but simultaneously takes me to different places—without my having to change hotel rooms.

Moving is another event that—in addition to being generally stressful—produces a change in routine. And it is not only a change in where one lives that can have this effect—it also can be caused by changing work locations.

A number of years ago a patient of mine—Jorge—decided to move his law practice to a more central location in town to expand his business. Both his psychiatrist and I cautioned Jorge about the potentially destabilizing effect that the move could have on his mood. Despite our reservations, he decided to go through with it.

Of course, we all knew that Jorge would eventually adjust to his new space and the changes in routine that went along with his move. And he did, fortunately without a full-blown mood episode. But for a while he had some symptoms that indicated he might be getting hypomanic—sleeping 5 rather than his usual 8 hours a night, having more energy than usual, and being more productive. That's why his psychiatrist made a minor change in his medication for a couple of months and I increased the frequency of our therapy sessions (just to be on the safe side) while he was getting used to his new situation.

Sometimes change is unavoidable. Other times, as in Jorge's case, one elects to make a change because of the anticipated benefits. However, for people who have bipolar disorder, change—particularly change in routine—can lead to mood instability. You and your partner need to keep this in mind as you make life decisions together.

Support Your Mate in Abstaining from Alcohol

Violet spent years self-medicating her bipolar II illness with alcohol. Pressured by her partner to "do something" about her drinking problem, she scheduled an appointment with me. After several months of therapy, Violet came to see the relationship between her drinking and her mood disorder. As she put it, "It really became clear when I was hypomanic—all I had to do is count the number of empty vodka bottles in the recycle bin."

As I explained in Chapter 2, substance abuse—particularly alcohol abuse—is extremely prevalent among people who have bipolar disorder, appearing at some time during the course of the illness in at least 60% of individuals who have the diagnosis. Because of this prevalence, drinking can be a major source of conflict between partners (see the dialogue between Ellen and Hayden at the beginning of this chapter).

Alcohol is commonly used by bipolar people to self-medicate both in manic and depressive episodes, although research indicates it's more commonly used during manic or mixed states. The substance can initially produce a euphoric or high feeling, but it's important to know that alcohol actually is a central nervous system *depressant*, so after the initial high has subsided it can deepen the despair of someone who is in a depression. Also, in that alcohol is disinhibiting and affects one's judgment, drinking can increase the risky, impulsive behavior that often occurs during manic, mixed, and hypomanic episodes. The amount of alcohol bipolar individuals consume can be a good barometer of where they are with respect to their illness, as it was for Violet.

Although there may be some differences in opinion about whether bipolar people who are stabilized can occasionally consume small amounts of alcohol, there is no question when it comes to those who are in mood episodes. **Bipolar individuals who are in mood episodes—whether depressed or manic—should not under any circumstances ingest alcoholic beverages.** As I discussed in Chapter 2, research shows that alcohol worsens and lengthens existing mood episodes (possibly, at least in part, because it compromises the efficacy of pharmacological treatments) and dramatically increases the risk of suicide.

Even for individuals with mild forms of bipolar disorder who are well stabilized, doctors caution about alcohol use, and many suggest that the best strategy really is to completely abstain from drinking. My own opinion on the subject, however, is somewhat mixed. As is true for most professionals who specialize in this area, over the years I have seen many patients whose disorders have been dramatically worsened by alcohol. On the other hand, though, I've also seen patients who have their bipolar disorder under control who are able to have an occasional alcoholic beverage without any adverse consequences.

Wanting to do everything I could to have good mood health, after I accepted my diagnosis of bipolar disorder I gave up drinking for over a decade. While abstaining from alcohol was something of a sacrifice, I thought (as many professionals do) it was necessary in order for me to have mood stability. In recent years, though, I've allowed alcohol back into my life in a limited way—drinking occasionally, moderately—and there haven't been any negative consequences.

My own experience actually highlights the two areas that should be assessed in relation to alcohol use:

1. Does your partner drink in a controlled manner—only in specific, limited circumstances, such as socially, and only in moderate or "normal" amounts?
2. Is your partner's mood or behavior impacted negatively by drinking?

Clearly people who binge drink or get drunk or require alcohol on a regular basis aren't drinking in a controlled manner and therefore shouldn't drink. In fact, a person who is drinking in one of these ways may well need help to quit (see the sidebar on page 191). As to alcohol's effects on your partner, monitoring mood and simultaneously keeping track of alcohol consumption can help provide answers to the second question.

Ian insisted that his drinking did not have any effect on his bipolar disorder. In fact, he told me, if anything, alcohol improved his mood, particularly when he was hypomanic. He maintained that a moderate amount of alcohol decreased the racy feeling he had when his mood would get too high and that it also made him less distractible and better able to focus. However, after he monitored his mood for a couple of months along with his alcohol intake, it became clear that Ian's drinking actually was having a negative, not a positive, effect on him: consistently, the day following his drinking, his mood would be depressed.

If your partner is reluctant to look at the effects of her drinking by monitoring, it's a likely bet that alcohol is playing too great a role in her life and/or is causing problems. In all probability, you will have to share your own observations on this with your mate to get her to look at the truth.

What can you do to help support your mate in giving up alcohol? There are a number of lifestyle changes that the two of you can make that will help your partner remain sober. Read on.

Remove Alcohol from Your Home

The first step in achieving abstinence (besides making a commitment to give up alcohol) is to remove alcoholic beverages from your home. Just as with other habits and addictive behaviors that people have a hard time changing (giving up cigarettes, losing weight), it will be much easier for your loved one to abstain if temptation is not in his face.

Obviously, if alcohol is no longer present in your home, you also will be limiting your drinking. If you do not have an alcohol problem yourself and enjoy a cocktail or glass of wine with dinner, you may find this restrictive. You may also find, though, that it's a sacrifice worth making for your mate, at least for the short term, until your partner has sobriety well under her belt. In fact, if you are willing to completely abstain from drinking—both in and out of the home—along with your loved one (again, at least until your spouse is secure in her nondrinking), this will help your mate immensely.

Avoid Places and People Associated with Drinking

It also will be harder for your mate to refrain from drinking if surrounded by others who are engaging in this behavior. This can become a bit tricky if alcohol has been central to your social life. Staying away from bars and clubs, at least initially (until being a nondrinker becomes second nature), will help your partner. The two of you also may find that some of the other couples you used to go out with are not compatible with your new alcohol-free lives. If you can, you may want to suggest forms of entertainment and activities that don't lend themselves to drinking, such as going to the movies, shopping, or playing a sport. If your friends are not interested or willing to participate in activities that don't include alcohol, and you and your spouse are committed to

If Your Partner Has an Alcohol Problem

Those who have bipolar disorder and alcohol abuse or dependence would be described as having a "dual diagnosis." Expert consensus agrees that individuals with a dual diagnosis *must* become abstinent from their substance of choice. If your partner has an alcohol problem, he or she can choose among several different effective methods for reaching this goal.

One route is a 12-step program like **Alcoholics Anonymous** (AA). AA is a self-help group that promotes abstinence, the only criterion for membership being the desire to stop drinking. In addition to attending meetings, members are given "sponsors"—individuals who have successfully been abstinent for a specified period of time—with whom they have frequent contact. Many AA meetings are designated as "open" (as opposed to "closed")—that is, open to those, like partners, who are close to the individual with the alcohol problem.

If your mate does not want to deal with his problem in a group setting, there is another possibility: he could have **individual therapy,** offered by many practitioners, that follows a 12-step model. Or your partner could do both; many of my dually diagnosed patients attend AA meetings along with having individual sessions with me. Cognitive– behavioral therapy (see Chapter 4)—administered individually or in a group format—has been shown to be helpful for some in achieving abstinence.

If your partner has developed alcohol dependence or has stopped drinking but still has frequent cravings or lapses, AA or therapy alone may not be sufficient. Several **medications** have been approved by the FDA specifically for treating alcohol dependence. None are addictive, and all can be administered on an outpatient basis.

If your mate has failed to achieve abstinence repeatedly, you both may have to consider the possibility that a more intensive, restrictive program is what's needed. Most **residential programs** span for 1 or 2 months or even longer. Many include a family therapy component as a necessary part of the treatment process. *If your partner needs a residential program, make sure that it deals with people who have dual diagnoses.* Your partner's doctor should be able to recommend a facility that's right for your mate.

an alcohol-free lifestyle, you may have to consider the possibility that these are no longer the people you should be spending your free time with. (Please know that I'm not saying this lightly. However, it's an issue that many couples have to face if they want to lead nondrinking lives.)

Consider a Self-Help Group

If your mate has trouble stopping drinking, another way you can support her in being abstinent is to attend open meetings of Alcoholics Anonymous (AA) together (see the sidebar on page 191). If, however, for whatever reason, your mate has decided to participate in a closed meeting of AA as her regular group, meaning you can't attend, you can still show your support—and possibly gain useful insights into your and your spouse's behavior—by going to an Alanon group. Alanon was expressly designed for family members and others who are close to people with alcohol problems. And as an added benefit, both AA and Alanon provide opportunities to interact with and potentially befriend individuals who are committed to nondrinking lifestyles.

Substance abuse: Recurrent, significant negative consequences from repeated use of the substance; does not meet the criteria for substance dependence.

Substance dependence: Repeated use of the substance results in the development of tolerance, withdrawal, and compulsive drug-taking/drug-seeking behavior.

In addition to alcohol, I've found in my practice that bipolar people may use street drugs or abuse prescription drugs to self-medicate and "manage" their moods. For example, some individuals try to reduce the raciness and anxiety that accompanies manic or mixed states with marijuana, or, alternatively, use stimulants like cocaine and amphetamines during mania or hypomania to achieve an even "higher high." People experiencing depressive episodes also may abuse stimulants (street or prescription—see the sidebar on page 193) because of their mood-elevating qualities. The methods used to treat alcohol disorders (see the sidebar on pages 191) have been modified so that they're useful in treating problems with street or prescription drugs too.

Prescription Stimulants, Caffeine, and Bipolar Disorder

Because attention-deficit/hyperactivity disorder (ADHD) can be confused with bipolar disorder, especially among children and adolescents, it's not usual to find a history of stimulant prescriptions (Ritalin, Adderall) among those diagnosed as bipolar. Stimulants may be warranted for some treatment-resistant bipolar depressions or for dual diagnoses of ADHD and bipolar disorder, but many physicians will otherwise avoid prescribing stimulants because of their high addictive potential and their ability to trigger or exacerbate mania and hypomania.

Unfortunately, those who were maintained on stimulants before a diagnosis of bipolar disorder was firmed up have often gotten used to the "lift" that these drugs induced, and when the stimulants are discontinued many turn to excessive caffeine use to try to duplicate the feeling. Even people who haven't been taking stimulants may try to combat the sedation that comes with many bipolar medications with large amounts of caffeine. Although caffeine probably is less dramatic than stimulant medication in its effects on mood, questions have emerged regarding the effects of the so-called "energy drinks"—beverages containing extraordinarily high amounts of caffeine—that have become popular in recent years.

Help Your Loved One Face and Resolve Conflicts

Research has shown that interpersonal conflict—particularly with one's spouse or other close family members—increases the likelihood that bipolar episodes will recur.

Dealing with Problems Together

Unresolved conflict increases stress, and stress, as I've discussed before, can trigger a mood episode (see the sidebar on page 195 for more on unresolved conflicts between your partner and other individuals). That's why it's so important for you and your partner to develop effective strategies to face and solve relationship problems together. Here are some tips for doing just that:

- Set aside time on a regular basis to talk, just the two of you, without any distractions.
- Clearly communicate what your concerns are.
- Try to stay calm—don't resort to shouting, screaming, swearing, or "hitting below the belt."
- Don't be accusatory. Use "I" rather than "You" statements.
- Keep the conversation on current issues—don't bring in situations from the past unless they are directly relevant to the present situation.
- Recognize that solving problems often requires compromise from each of the parties involved (see page 195 for more on problem solving).

Know Your Partner's "Hot Topics"

Earlier in this chapter I talked about identifying trigger situations that cause mood fluctuations. There also are "trigger conversations," that is, topics of conversation that tend to provoke mood shifts in your mate. I'm not referring here to conversations that focus on solving relationship or other problems, like in the previous section. These are specific topics that generally tend to get a negative emotional reaction from your mate.

Your partner's sensitive topics can include things that are understandably difficult to discuss (such as a traumatic event), or, on the other hand, they may seem insignificant or even silly to you (like your mate's hairstyle), but still get a big reaction from your spouse. Use the space below to list five of your mate's trigger topics:

My Partner's Hot Topics

1. _____
2. _____
3. _____
4. _____
5. _____

It's important to know which specific topics are likely to set your mate off so that you can steer clear of these sensitive areas (unless, of course, it's an urgent situation that must be dealt with immediately). Again, let me emphasize, do not bring up these subjects on your own. Instead, wait for your partner to introduce the topic; chances are he'll do so when he's ready to deal with it.

A hot topic of mine is related to new technology. Unlike many people, I don't want the latest cell phone or notebook computer—actually, it's not just that I don't want these things; the idea of trading in my current ones for new ones makes me *anxious*. (I think it has something to do with being a bit "technologically challenged," but I could be wrong.) If my husband even broaches the subject with me—"Honey, don't you think it's time that you traded in your _____ for a new _____?"—I will react in a not pleasant manner. And if he continues to push the subject, we're definitely headed for a fight. So he's learned to wait

The Four Steps of Problem Solving

1. **Identify** the problem.
2. Come up with alternative **solutions**.
3. **Choose** a solution.
4. Put the solution into **action**.

Does Your Partner Have an Unresolved Conflict?

- Is your mate no longer communicating with someone who was once close because of an ongoing relationship problem?

- Does your partner always get tense or uptight when interacting with a particular individual with whom she has strong ties? Does she try to avoid contact with that person?

- Does your loved one tell you that he has recurrent, disturbing dreams about someone who played a significant role in his life?

- Has your mate told you about a past relationship that she has never really gotten over?

- Has your partner lost someone close to him but has never gone through the process of grieving?

---

for me to bring up the topic (which, coincidentally, I recently have, regarding my computer—it's finally time for a new one).

Once your mate has broached a difficult topic, don't assume that things will necessarily go smoothly from that point on. If you see that the conversation and your mate's mood are taking a wrong turn—your partner is becoming agitated or tearful, for example—my advice is to say something like "Why don't we talk about this more later?" and then change the topic to deescalate the situation. If your partner insists on continuing to discuss the topic in his overemotional state ("No, I want to talk about it now!"), stay calm, stay quiet, and just *listen*. Don't react. At this point your mate probably is looking for a fight—don't fall into this trap.

Conflict Arising from Misperceptions

Bipolar people often tend to personalize and feel easily slighted by the actions of others. Whereas some people would overlook a comment or situation and could readily push it aside, those with bipolar disorder may intently focus on it—become almost riveted by it—and then overreact to the perceived wrong. That's the situation Christine found herself in.

> *Christine:* I can't believe that my sister didn't invite us to her party. What an insult! I can't even look at her after that.
>
> *Bill:* She said the party was just for friends, not family members.
>
> *Christine:* I don't care. We're really close, and I should have been there.
>
> *Bill:* But she didn't invite your sister Ann, either.
>
> *Christine:* Well, two wrongs don't make a right! I'm surprised Ann isn't bent out of shape about this too.
>
> *Bill:* That's because Ann understands that there's a time and place to be with relatives and that this wasn't one of them.
>
> *Christine:* Ann isn't as close to Mandy as I am.
>
> *Bill:* That's true. But the same principle applies. How would

it be for Mandy to invite one sister to the party but not the other?

Christine: She could have invited both of us.

Bill: And what if she had you and your sister to the party but didn't invite your folks? How do you think that would be?

Christine: Not good, I guess.

Bill: So this really isn't *about you*. It's about the fact that Mandy wanted to have a small gathering of just her friends, not have all of us—her family—there too.

Bill did a good job of showing Christine that her sister's behavior wasn't a personal slight. But what if Christine still didn't let the situation go, even after Bill made his case?

Christine: I'm still hurt.

Bill: I don't think she meant to hurt you.

Christine: It doesn't matter if she meant it. A hurt is a hurt.

Bill: I think if she knew how much it would affect you she might have handled the situation differently. She might have talked to you beforehand.

Christine: Well, it doesn't matter now. It's too late.

Bill: Why don't you tell her how you feel?

Christine: What good will that do?

Bill: It might help the two of you get past this.

Christine: I don't know.

Bill: Well, it can't hurt to give it a try.

Christine: Maybe. I'll think about it.

Bill: Don't think about it; just do it.

Christine: Okay, okay, I guess you're right.

Here Bill was able to persuade Christine to share her feelings about not being invited to the party by her sister. The ability to communicate feelings—both positive and negative (when appropriate)—is a very important factor in keeping relationships healthy.

As I've outlined in this chapter, there are many things—besides being consistent with medication—that your mate can do, often with your help, to be proactive and prevent mood episodes from recurring. If you find, however, that the pendulum begins to swing despite these efforts, see the next two chapters, which offer lots of specific suggestions as to what you and your partner can do.

8

Strategies for Dealing with the Ups Together

It's 3:00 A.M., and Martha has been riveted to the computer screen looking at items on eBay for the past 4 hours. Her husband, Peter, knows her signs of hypomania, and she's exhibiting them all—sleeping less, having a lot more energy than usual, and being obsessed with home shopping. If they don't take action now, he also knows she could get worse fast.

Peter: *It's three o'clock in the morning, and you're still sitting here shopping.*

Martha: *I'm not tired.*

Peter: *But you know how important it is to get the right amount of sleep.*

Martha: *I don't seem to need as much sleep lately.*

Peter: *Exactly. You know what that means. It means you are beginning to get up there again.*

Martha: *Well, I like being, as you call it, "up there." I'm having a good time.*

Peter: *Your good times land us in trouble. The last time you were manic you racked up $20,000 in credit card bills, and it took us nearly 2 years to pay it off.*

Martha: *I won't let it get out of hand this time.*

Peter: *The only way to make sure it doesn't get out of hand is to take steps to stop your mood from getting even higher. That includes going to bed at your usual time and giving up the shopping. You've got to get back to your normal routine.*

Martha: *Okay, I'll go to bed at my normal time, but I'm not completely giving up shopping.*

Peter: *Well, if you don't, we'll have to go to Plan B, the one we laid out in our agreement. No credit cards, no checks, no ATM card—you know you won't like that.*

Martha: *You're so controlling!*

Peter: *I'm just concerned for your health and for our future.*

Martha: *Okay, fine. You win. And I hope you're happy—I was just outbid on something I really wanted to buy.*

Mania can have a devastating effect on people's lives. I use the plural *lives* here because manic episodes don't affect only the individuals who have them; they impact those close by as well. That includes, first and foremost, you and any children you have. It also includes friends, relatives, coworkers, and employers—anyone who plays an important role in your partner's life.

Manic behavior can infiltrate and wreak havoc in multiple arenas—relationships, work, finances, spirituality, and physical health, to name a few. And, possibly even more important, its impact can be felt long after an episode is over. Divorce, unemployment, bankruptcy, incarceration, illness, and even in some cases death are among the tragic, but unfortunately not uncommon, consequences of these episodes.

As you know from earlier chapters in this book, the nature of bipolar illness is that it is recurrent. So even with all the best preventive measures in place, your mate's mood may elevate significantly and become a cause for concern at times. That's why you should read this chapter even if you and your partner are taking all the precautions available to avoid recurrences of mania. You want to be prepared for the worst, especially in light of the potentially catastrophic consequences manic episodes can bring.

Hypomania and mania very frequently emerge when people are not taking their mood-stabilizing medications as prescribed (see Chapter 6), but they can also be triggered by environmental circumstances or biological/physical factors, as I've explained in previous chapters, some of which people have control over and others over which they have no control. Something as seemingly innocuous as a change in daily routine or a busy period at work can set off an episode in certain individuals. Over time some people's "chemistry" changes in such a way that it alters the efficacy of the medication they are taking and "breakthrough" mood episodes appear. Even daylight savings time or the change of seasons can bring on a mood shift toward mania.

Besides making all the preventive efforts described in Chapter 7, the best way to ward off unexpected attacks of mania is to *identify potential episodes very early on.* Early identification opens up the possibility of early intervention, which can keep your loved one's mild mood change from blossoming into a full-blown manic episode, the type of mood problem that can bring on the devastating consequences I mentioned before. Therefore, this chapter focuses first on how to spot your partner's early warning signs of hypomania/mania and what to do when you've identified them. Next, in the event you and your partner can't circumvent a full-blown manic episode, the chapter maps out a plan for helping your mate through this while also paying attention to your own physical and emotional needs.

How Do I Know When My Partner Is Becoming Manic?

Hypomanic and manic episodes generally don't come completely out of the blue. Usually there are warning signs indicating they're on the way. Although the specific signs can vary quite a bit among individuals, they tend to be pretty consistent across episodes for a particular person. For instance, I know my mood is on the upswing when I require less sleep to feel rested (typically about a 2-hour decrease in sleep per night), have more energy throughout the day, am more jovial than usual, and find that my perception of my surroundings is more sensitive—for example, colors seem brighter and bright lights seem more intense.

I know these things about myself probably, at least in part, because I'm a psychologist. Being an observer of human behavior—including my own—gives me the ability to step outside myself and look at my thoughts, feelings, and behaviors fairly objectively so that I know where I am with respect to my mood. And then, being aware of my own idiosyncratic early warning signs of hypomania, I can take steps to intervene before things get out of hand.

However, I know that this ability does not come readily to everyone, and in fact my bipolar patients in particular often find they have trouble stepping outside themselves and seeing their behavior in an objective way. Since they're not always aware of when they are headed for a mood episode, we work on their self-observation skills in therapy. But I also think it helps when my patients' partners can identify the signs of an impending mood swing too. You can provide valuable feedback to your mate and/or, if necessary, to the doctor so that quick action potentially can nip an episode in the bud.

Do you remember Sam, the man I described at the beginning of Chapter 6 who was cutting his pills in half? Sam, in his wife's words, was "agitated, argumentative, and slightly 'paranoid,'" all symptoms that his wife knew were early warning signs of mania. When I asked her to elaborate on what she meant, she said, "He's easily annoyed by little things and seems to want to pick fights with me." She then went on to say, "He's very suspicious of other people's motives, not taking what they do or say at face value, even people we've known for a long time." When I asked her if there was anything else she noticed that concerned her, she replied that Sam was waking up earlier than usual, by 1 to 2 hours.

Sam's Early Warning Signs of Mania

- Easily annoyed
- Picks fights
- Suspicious
- Sleeping less

Marilee's husband, Tom, saw several changes in his wife's behavior that concerned him. He said, "She's drinking wine with dinner pretty much every night," rather than her usual one or two times a week. He also commented that Marilee was spending money "like water," not on big things but still enough to make a dent in the family's budget. She was talking faster and joking around a lot, two behaviors that Tom knew meant she was on the way "up." When I asked him if he had noticed any other changes, he said Marilee had been staying up later than usual to work on projects, like scrapbooking and cleaning out their closets.

Marilee's Early Warning Signs of Mania

- Increased drinking
- Increased shopping
- Talking faster
- Acting silly and joking around
- Going to bed later
- Increased productivity

Take a look at the items in the list on the next page. Although people are unique in the particular constellation of early warning signs they exhibit (like Sam and Marilee), I've tried to be very inclusive here so that you should be able to find the ones that apply to your mate. I've also left room at the bottom for other signs you've observed that aren't listed.

Especially if your mate has been participating in cognitive–behavioral therapy or another form of therapy that teaches people to recognize their own early warning signs, your partner should participate in the identification process. You two can fill out the form together, or you can do so independently and then compare to see where you agree. If your partner hasn't been in therapy that works on such identification, you can encourage her to reflect on past mood episodes to list warning signs.

If your mate has had very few hypomanic or manic episodes, it may be difficult for you to pinpoint the specific symptoms that occur at the very beginning of a mood swing. In all likelihood you didn't realize there was a problem until you were in the thick of it. And by

Early Warning Signs of Mania

Circle all of the items that apply to your mate. Remember, for an item to count as a warning sign, it must represent a change from your mate's usual behavior during periods of normal mood.

Easily irritated or annoyed

Seems to be looking for fights (verbal)

Very anxious, edgy, or uptight

Very upbeat

More self-confident

Bragging about him- or herself

More assertive

Wanting to travel

Spending more money

Consuming more alcohol

Consuming more caffeine

Has big plans—wants to start a new business, move to another state, etc.

More outgoing or gregarious

Silly or joking around a lot

Singing or humming out loud

Walking with a spring to his or her step or faster than usual

Sleeping less

Very energetic

Exercising more than usual

More sexual

Absorbed by projects (work or hobbies)

Driving faster or more aggressively

Very creative

Thinking seems accelerated

Easily distracted

More optimistic

More talkative or talking faster

Perceives others as walking (talking, driving, etc.) more slowly than they should

Suspicious or "paranoid"

Finds "hidden meanings" in things that aren't apparent to others

More religious

Questioning the meaning of life or consumed by other existential/philosophical concerns

Other behaviors: _____

_____

_____

_____

then I'm sure you were more involved in addressing the situation than in looking back to identify the early indicators of the mood swing. Now, however, in retrospect, you can review your partner's episodes and see whether a particular pattern of changes occurred early on for each of them.

I used the plural *changes* quite intentionally, by the way. Any individual item by itself may not indicate that your partner is becoming hypomanic or manic, but when you see a *cluster* of symptoms together, you're more likely to be seeing the early warning signs of an episode. For example, being more sexual, shopping more, or being silly by themselves may not be a cause for concern, but *together* they suggest a mood shift.

Now that you've reviewed the list and determined which signs relate to your spouse, take a few minutes and write them on the form on the next page.

What Do I Do When I See Early Warning Signs?

Now that you know your partner's early warning signs of mania, what actions should you take? First, talk to your significant other about what you've observed. This isn't always easy, of course. It needs to be done delicately so that your mate doesn't get defensive and angry and decide to completely discount what you have to say. Also, keep in mind that a lot of people enjoy their hypomanic or manic states, so your partner may be invested in "pretending" (denying) that this is not what's going on.

When Tom broached the subject with Marilee, she disagreed with what he had to say. And when Isabel tried to talk to Sam about her concerns, he snapped at her. How could these people have approached their spouses so that the message would be taken more seriously?

One thing you definitely don't want to do is to say, "I think you're getting manic [or hypomanic] again." A remark like this, on the face of it, may not seem offensive. I guarantee you, though, that it will make most individuals who are on the way up get angry or slough off the comment. It is better to approach the situation by gently pointing out specific things you've noticed. Let's see how Tom could have handled this with Marilee:

My Partner's Early Warning Signs of Mania

List at least three changes that appear together (during the same period of time) at the very beginning of your partner's hypomanic or manic episodes.

Early Warning Sign #1:

_____

_____

Early Warning Sign #2:

_____

_____

Early Warning Sign #3:

_____

_____

Early Warning Sign #4:

_____

_____

Early Warning Sign #5:

_____

_____

From *When Someone You Love Is Bipolar* by Cynthia G. Last. Copyright 2009 by Cynthia G. Last.

Tom: I've noticed some changes lately that have me a bit concerned.

Marilee: Like what?

Tom: Like you've been drinking and shopping more than usual, not so bad that it's out of hand, but I'm worried it might become a problem again.

Marilee: Tom, you're making more of this than there is. I've just gotten into the habit of drinking wine with dinner—a lot of people do that. And, as for the shopping, you know I've lost weight recently. I really do need new clothes.

Tom: And what about the giggling all the time? You know what that means.

Marilee: So I'm a happy person, big deal. I enjoy life. I like wine, I like shopping, I like to laugh and have a good time.

Tom: I like that you're happy. I just don't want you to get too happy, so you end up like you were last spring. Remember how bad that got? And remember the month before you got that way you were acting the same way you're acting now?

Marilee: No, I don't remember that. I don't get what you're saying.

Tom: I'm saying that we need to pay attention to the little changes now, before they become a big problem.

Marilee: You know, you worry too much. But if it makes you feel better, I'll talk to my doctor.

As you can see in this example, Tom's persistence paid off. Although Marilee acted like she was appeasing him ("If it makes you feel better ... "), the end result was the one Tom was looking for.

Not everyone, of course, will react this way. You might have to have a conversation like the one Tom had with Marilee a number of times before successfully getting the message across. Or you may need to pull out the agreement the two of you should make for exactly this purpose. The behavioral contract described later in this chapter specifies the warning signs for hypomania or mania and what the two of you will do in the event that they arise.

Sometimes, though, no matter how hard you try, your efforts to help are met with resistance and denial. In a case like this you may have to communicate with your mate's doctor (by making a phone call, by sending a letter, an e-mail, or a fax, or by accompanying your partner to her appointment) to apprise the doctor of what's been going on. Although your partner may get annoyed with you now for "taking

Talking to Your Partner during the Early Warning Sign Period

Don't ...

- *Respond to the irritability.* Ignore—don't personalize and react to—comments that stem from your partner's edginess (even if they are directed at you), like complaints, criticisms, and sarcastic remarks.
- *Bring up touchy subjects.* Avoid topics and questions that raise issues your mate typically (even when in a normal mood state) finds difficult to address—raising them now would be even more agitating.
- *Argue, even if you're right.* Engaging your partner in a heated debate will increase his emotionality and worsen symptoms. Besides, you won't win—you're far more likely to succeed with logic (see "Do," below).
- *Be a "Chatty Cathy."* Too much conversation can be overstimulating to your mate. As much as you can, try to keep your time together relatively quiet and relaxing.

Do ...

- *Speak calmly and slowly.* Raising your voice or speaking very rapidly (even if it's because of positive feelings you're having) is likely to increase your partner's excitability and possibly worsen symptoms.
- *Use logic.* Most people can be rational during the early stages of an episode and will respond positively to your prompts to do so. For example, if your mate is feeling a "right now" urge to spend too much money on something, you might point out that it's often helpful to contemplate large purchases for a while ("Why don't you sleep on it?") before "taking the plunge."
- *Give your mate breathing room.* At this stage of an episode your mate is not so ill that he needs a constant companion. Let your partner have time alone (provided it's not being used for destructive, rather than constructive, purposes).
- *Problem solve together.* Things that your mate normally would handle easily on her own can feel overwhelming during the early stages of mania. Help your partner to clearly delineate the problem(s), generate viable solutions, then choose and implement a strategy that's likely to work (see Chapter 7 for more on problem solving).

over," she may later thank you for taking the steps to ensure that the illness doesn't progress.

The Early Intervention Plan

By identifying a mild hypomanic state early on, your partner and you can take measures to try to prevent the mood from escalating into a full-fledged manic state. This is known as "early intervention."

The following measures are those I've found most useful in preventing a mild, hypomanic mood from progressing to one that's more severe. Most of these strategies have been found effective in research studies as well.

1. *Institute whatever means are necessary to ensure that your mate gets sufficient sleep.* As you know from the preceding chapter, decreased sleep, a common symptom of hypomania, can worsen a mood episode. If your mate is trying to get to sleep but having trouble doing so, encourage her to use the sleep hygiene tips in Chapter 7 and/ or, if necessary, to discuss with the doctor the possibility of prescription sleep medication. But if your partner *doesn't want* to go to sleep, you may have to pull out all the stops because it's absolutely imperative that you do whatever you can to persuade your partner to return to her regular bedtime. One strategy that may work is to put the onus on yourself, saying something like "I really need a lot of sleep right now because of my own schedule, and it's hard for me to sleep when you're awake and active; won't you come to bed with me so we can both get a good night's sleep?" Or, you may try using a negotiating tactic, such as "If you do this, then I'll do _____." Finally, you can always point to the behavioral contract (see page 225), the written agreement where your mate indicated she would make sleep a priority in just such a situation as this.

2. *Encourage your partner to avoid prolonged sun exposure.* Prolonged exposure to bright, white light is a treatment for depression and, like many treatments for depression, can precipitate the development of mania. Suggest that your mate avoid activities involving *excessive* sun exposure while having early warning signs. For instance, instead of spending the day at the beach or lounging by the pool, which typically

involves numerous hours outside, suggest a 1-hour bike ride or a game of tennis. Or better yet, take the bicycling or tennis *inside*, by means of a stationary bike or indoor tennis court.

3. *Stick to your family's normal routine.* As you know from Chapter 7, changes in routine can further destabilize your mate's mood. Here's where you might be able to make a significant difference. When you see the early warning signs of mania, immediately ask yourself whether the family routine has slipped. Have mealtimes become more irregular? Have any little changes been made in the way you two go about your day? If so, do everything you can to change them back. For things you do together, your spouse may have little choice but to follow your lead. If you're the cook in the family, adhere strictly to scheduled mealtimes. If you're not the cook, bring home a take-out meal at the scheduled time so your bipolar partner doesn't have control over the time meals are served. Even for those parts of the daily routine that don't usually involve you, you may be able to help restore stability. If your partner's mode of transportation to and from work has changed, see if you can find a way to make sure it doesn't take more time than it used to or cause more stress. If the train schedule has changed unfavorably, are there any carpooling possibilities? Could you two share a car and alternate driving each other to work? Try to keep to your normal schedule as much as possible, particularly when your mate is showing early warning signs.

4. *Avoid excessive stimulation.* Increased stimulation of any type—social, sexual, intellectual—carries with it the possibility of escalating mood. Now is not the time to throw a big party or encourage your partner to start working on a new business venture. Undoubtedly you know your partner well enough to find subtle ways to discourage any ideas she has that might be overstimulating. Whenever possible, avoid rejecting your partner's ideas outright; instead try using your own current limitations as an out. You could say you're just too busy with work right now to plan a party and would prefer to put it off for a while. You could express interest in a project proposed by your partner but suggest first steps, such as research, that will forestall any hasty investments of time, energy, or money.

5. *Increase physical activity.* Your partner may benefit from increasing exercise and other forms of physical activity during this period—to decrease his overall level of anxiety and/or use up some of the excess energy. To encourage this, you might start suggesting a long

walk after dinner or offer to get up early for a game of tennis. Would your partner appreciate your offer of a ride to the health club with you or on your way to another place?

6. *Keep stress to a minimum.* Consider shouldering "more of the load" while your mate is experiencing early warning signs. Is this too big a burden on you? You do have to think of yourself too (see Chapter 10). It may be worthwhile having help waiting in the wings for just such occasions if you can manage it. Also, do your best to avoid conflict with your mate during this time (which may be difficult since mildly elevated moods can include irritability too; see the sidebar on page 208). Antistress methods, like relaxation techniques, yoga, and meditation, may help as well (see Resources).

7. *Persuade your mate to postpone making any major life decisions.* Since hypomania can impair judgment, your partner should not be making important decisions until her mood has returned to normal. See some of the suggestions in item 4, above, for how to go about doing this. Here too, you may have to be creatively subtle to encourage your spouse to postpone important decisions.

8. *If you can identify a trigger situation, take steps to remove it or mitigate its impact.* For example, if your mate has been working extra hours, encourage him to reduce his workload (if possible) right away. If starting a new medication is associated with the elevated mood, make sure the doctor is aware of this so that she can make the appropriate changes.

9. *Keep in close contact with your mate.* By checking in periodically, you can keep abreast of any further fluctuations in your partner's mood. For instance, the two of you can agree to touch base on the telephone at noon every day just so you can be aware of how your mate is doing. However, please don't take this suggestion as indicating you should be in *constant* contact with your partner—"hovering" can be annoying and may increase your mate's level of agitation. It also sends the message that you feel your mate is not going to be okay, which can increase your partner's own level of anxiety about her condition and inadvertently make her worse.

10. *Make sure the rest of the treatment team is aware of the current situation.* Check with your mate to find out when his next medication and therapy appointments are scheduled—if not in the near future, encourage your mate to move them up. Also consider increasing the frequency of medication/therapy sessions just for the present time.

What If the Symptoms Escalate Too Quickly for the Early Intervention Plan?

Sometimes people go from having warning signs to full-blown mania in a very short period of time, such as a few hours or a couple of days. In a situation like this you won't have much time to communicate your observations to your mate or for the two of you to put an early intervention plan into place. Moreover, if your partner becomes severely manic and has no insight into how seriously ill she currently is, it's unlikely that talking with her about it will get you very far (in fact, it's possible that this will actually make matters worse by aggravating your mate). Instead, **you will need to contact your mate's psychiatrist right away** so that he can determine what actions need to be taken.

If the doctor judges the situation to be a true medical emergency, he may instruct you to admit your mate to a hospital immediately (see the sidebar on the facing page for more on this). But in all likelihood, the doctor will want to see your partner as soon as possible, at which time he will evaluate what medication changes need to be implemented. Alternatively, your spouse's physician may choose to call in a prescription for a medication to a pharmacy right away—even before meeting face-to-face with your partner—so that your mate can get started immediately on it.

The changes your loved one's doctor may make could include any or all of the following:

- Adding a new medication (or medications) to your partner's existing drug regimen
- Substituting a new medication for one your mate has—up till this point—been maintained on
- Increasing the dose (or doses) of your mate's current medication

Some medications used to stabilize manic patients take effect very rapidly, while others take days or weeks to work. Therefore, your mate's physician may prescribe two (or more) drugs, one to help immediately in suppressing manic behavior but to be used only for the short term, the other to be used on a more long-term basis but requiring time to become effective. (See Chapter 4 for more detailed information on the drugs typically used in the acute management of mania.)

Psychiatric Hospitals: What to Consider

- Is my partner's doctor affiliated with the hospital? If not, why does she recommend this particular hospital?
- Does the hospital take my form of insurance? What, if any, are likely to be my costs?
- Can I take a tour of the facility prior to admitting my partner?
- If my partner has a dual diagnosis (see Chapter 7), does the hospital offer concurrent treatment for alcohol/substance abuse?
- What experience does the hospital have in treating bipolar disorder?
- If the hospital is not local, how will I transport my partner to the facility in the event he or she needs to be admitted?

If your mate's mania worsens, and he is judged to be an imminent danger to himself or someone else, a short-term hospital stay may be necessary. ***Have a hospital in place before you need it***, so you don't have to deal with the logistics of where your mate will be going when you have a crisis on your hands. Your mate's doctor may be affiliated with one or more psychiatric hospitals in your area; ask the doctor to specify a preferred facility in the event a hospitalization is needed. *Make sure you have the name, address, and phone number of the hospital close at hand* and that you have a good idea of where it's located (and how to get there).

How Can I Keep My Partner and Family Safe during a Manic Episode?

As you know from Chapter 1, a characteristic of hypomania and mania is involvement in situations that have a high likelihood of negative—often painful—consequences. People in elevated mood states frequently exercise poor judgment and act impulsively, behaving in a way that ends up adversely affecting themselves and the ones they love. The circumstances that tend to be associated with high-risk behavior usually involve money, driving, sex, and substance use/abuse, or, if psychotic features are present, behavior that occurs in response to delusions or hallucinations.

When your mate is thinking about doing something risky or dangerous, the first thing you may want to try is to discuss the potential negative consequences and point out better alternatives. If your partner has bipolar II disorder (and, therefore, is experiencing a hypomanic episode) or is only mildly manic (see the scale in Chapter 7, pages 174–175), this may work. If she is more severely ill or if this strategy just doesn't work, you may be able to persuade your partner to avoid participating in potentially problematic situations by exerting the appropriate amount of pressure. The key word here is *appropriate*— you want to make sure you don't push too hard or your partner may end up rebelling and acting in even more potentially dangerous ways. (See the driving example on pages 215–216 for how to go about this.)

Other times, though, no matter what you do or say, your loved one will be determined to do something that could cause him, and quite possibly you too, serious trouble down the road. That's when you need to take more extreme actions, like the ones I talk about in the next few pages. (If you have a behavioral contract, many of these safety measures will be included there.)

Money

Excessive spending—shopping sprees, gambling, investing in risky ventures—is a manic behavior that can cause serious problems for bipolar individuals and their families.

What can you do to protect your mate and yourself? The very first thing is to have a list of financial institutions and account numbers for bank accounts, credit cards, etc. Then restrict your partner's access to money and valuables by taking the following actions:

- Ask your partner to surrender all *credit cards* or limit use to just one card that has a low (well below your financial means) spending limit.
- Have your mate turn over *ATM cards* and *blank checks*.
- Consider the use of "*direct deposit*" for your spouse's paychecks. This way, she won't be able to go to the bank and cash them.
- Set up *savings accounts, money market accounts*, etc., to require

both of your signatures for withdrawals. In other words, change the required signatures from "or" to "and."

- Give your mate *pocket money* (small amounts of cash) on a regular basis, such as $25 every day or two, rather than larger amounts less frequently.
- Do not let your mate have free access to *safety deposit boxes*, in-home *safes*, or any other repositories for valuables.
- Watch out for Internet and other forms of *home shopping*. Even though you've taken away the credit cards, your partner may have previously saved/stored credit card information with his account (for example, having a PayPal account on eBay).

Driving

Mania can lead people to drive at dangerously high speeds and very aggressively, tailgating and weaving in and out of different lanes. "Road rage" is common, as is drinking and driving.

If your partner's driving has become hazardous to herself and others, you need to speak frankly with her about the problem and come up with a solution that will protect your mate (as well as the other people she may inadvertently injure through her recklessness). Frequently this solution entails your stepping in and doing the driving— that is, just until your spouse's mood returns to normal. That's the situation Karen found herself in with her husband, Tyler:

Karen: I'm really worried about the way you've been driving.

Tyler: What do you mean? My driving is fine. In fact, it's never been better.

Karen: You're going way over the speed limit and running lights too.

Tyler: Everyone else is driving too slow. I like to get where I want to go, not lollygag around like the rest of these senior citizens.

Karen: But what if you get pulled over? You're already in danger of having your license suspended.

Tyler: I won't get pulled over.

Karen: That's what you said the other times, and now you're just one ticket away from not being able to drive.

Tyler: So what? If I can't drive, I won't.

Karen: But think about it; really think about it. Picture what it would be like to have to rely on someone else every time you need or want to go somewhere. Having your mobility hampered like that, I think it would really bother you.

Tyler: It might piss me off.

Karen: Right. So why don't we make sure that doesn't happen? Let me do the driving just for a little while, until you feel less of a need for speed.

By pointing out the potential negative consequences of his actions, Karen was able to get her husband to hand over the car keys. But what if Tyler didn't react this way? What if he said no to Karen? What could she have done in that case? As you'll see, Karen responds by bringing out "the big guns," showing Tyler how truly catastrophic his behavior could be, not only to himself but to their entire family.

Tyler: I'm not giving you the car keys. No way!

Karen: Well, I'm not going to be a passenger in this car with you driving this fast.

Tyler: Fine. I'll drop you off at home, and you can take your own car. I don't need to have you hounding me anyway.

Karen: I'm not "hounding" you; I'm trying to save your life. But if you insist on risking yours, that's one thing. I'm not risking mine too. Do you want our kids to grow up without us? Is that what you want for them?

Tyler: All right, already. I've heard enough. You want to do the driving, go ahead.

If Karen still couldn't get Tyler to relinquish the keys, even after this interchange, she may have had to resort to physically removing them from his possession, like when he was sleeping or involved in some other activity, and then at a later point explain what she had done and why she'd done it.

If you have to take away the keys, you can expect your partner to get very angry with you for your "controlling" behavior (if he doesn't, you're lucky), to which you may respond, "I'm doing this because I love you and I'm concerned for your safety." If you've set up a behavioral contract as described on page 225, you can point to the contract and show your mate his signature, indicating that he's agreed to turn the car keys over to you at the first signs of a manic episode.

Alcohol

As I explained in previous chapters, it's very common for bipolar people to abuse alcohol when in mood episodes, particularly during hypomanic/manic/mixed periods. This is a very troubling behavior because it has such serious consequences, including increasing the length and severity of mood episodes (possibly, at least in part, because alcohol interferes with the effectiveness of bipolar medications) and increasing the risk of suicide. If those deterrents aren't enough, alcohol intoxication can increase impulsivity and hamper judgment, which means your mate is even more likely to engage in high-risk behaviors when inebriated.

What can you do to help your partner abstain from alcohol? In addition to following the suggestions in Chapter 7, your greatest likelihood of success rests on making sure that your mate is being medicated properly for the current mood episode. *Reducing the manic symptoms should also lessen the urge to drink,* which will make it easier for your partner not to imbibe.

How can you know if your partner is being medicated *properly*? By this time you should have a physician in place that you and your loved one trust to prescribe medicine for your partner (if you don't, see Chapter 4 for guidelines for finding one). Making the doctor aware of the current situation as soon as possible (once you've seen evidence of mania) is vital so that the psychiatrist can make the appropriate changes in your spouse's medicine right away.

The second half of making sure your mate is being medicated properly is to see that your partner is following the doctor's orders to the letter. Unfortunately, your mate may refuse to do this or may hide noncompliance from you and the doctor because she enjoys the mania.

If you've discovered or you suspect that your mate is lying to you about taking his medication as prescribed, you may want to ask him to take it in front of you. You might tell your mate you want to do this just to put your own mind at ease, which is considerably softer than saying something like "Because I don't trust you!" If this doesn't work and your partner still refuses to adhere to his medication regimen, the doctor may decide to deliver the medication intramuscularly (by injection) or determine that a hospitalization is necessary to ensure your loved one's safety while he is being noncompliant.

Infidelity

It's not unusual for people in manic episodes to experience a heightened sense of sexuality. This by itself isn't necessarily a cause for concern. The problem is that during mania an increased libido doesn't occur by itself; it typically gets paired with gregariousness, poor judgment, and impulsivity, which together can trigger sexual behavior with far-reaching negative consequences.

The most obvious damage from infidelity is, of course, the effects it has on your relationship, which I discuss in Chapter 10. But there are other potential adverse outcomes, including the risk of sexually transmitted disease and pregnancy if impulsivity leads your partner to have unprotected sex. Mania also compromises your partner's judgment; people in mania's throes may choose inappropriate or dangerous sexual partners, sharing intimacies with a boss, a brother- or sister-in-law, or someone met in an Internet chat room, through an "escort" or "dating" service, or at an unsavory night spot.

These examples are not intended to frighten you. Not everyone who experiences mania becomes hypersexual. Even those whose libido does increase do not all engage in extramarital relationships; for many people their basic values prevail despite the effects of mania. And not all extramarital relations have catastrophic consequences.

Still, I'm sure you'd rather spare both of you the potential fallout of infidelity. Here, as with all other risky behavior associated with mania, the best way to protect your spouse from doing something now that she will regret later is to make sure her medication is adjusted at the very earliest signs of a mood problem. The sooner your partner's mood can be stabilized, the less room there will be for making unsound choices.

The other thing I advise you to do is to step up the check-ins with your mate (see point 9 in the Early Intervention Plan on page 211). By checking in more frequently you may be able to head off a problem before it actually gets to "the danger point." Of course, if your mate is severely manic and you've had to take away the car keys, there will be less chance for him to get into trouble just because of the sheer logistics involved. (However, don't be completely lulled into a false sense of security. Just because your spouse doesn't have access to his own car doesn't mean he can't find other ways to get around.)

Caring for the Children

I would be remiss if I didn't discuss the potential negative effects of mania on your children. On the positive side, even when your spouse is ill, there's another parent—you—available to attend to your children's emotional and physical needs. The fact that it's you may not always seem like good news when you're wrapped up in giving your mate the extra attention she needs at this time, on top of taking on the parenting responsibilities for both you and your partner. But perhaps you can gain some peace of mind from knowing that—at the end of the day— you are still there for your children.

Unfortunately, if your mate is very ill, he may be unable to care for the children. Although still physically present, your partner may be emotionally "removed" from the children, preoccupied with other things. He also may no longer be up to the active aspects of child rearing, such as providing meals, making sure the kids have clean clothes, and driving them to school.

And what about the emotional effects of having a bipolar parent on the children? Your children may feel frightened by the unfamiliar and possibly bizarre way their mother or father is acting. They most likely will feel a sense of loss because of your partner's being unable to be there for them as before. Your children may be embarrassed when others—like their friends—are able to observe your loved one's inappropriate or unusual behavior. They may be angry that they are the ones who have a parent who has an illness. (See Chapter 10 for how to talk to your child about your spouse's illness and how to seek professional help for your youngster, if needed; also, see Resources for a book for children who have a bipolar parent, "The Bipolar Bear Family.")

If your partner is very severely ill, you need to consider the possibility that her extremely poor judgment, marked impulsivity, or delusions or hallucinations could endanger your children. If this is the case, **either your children or your mate should be removed from the home.** If, considering an extreme example, your significant other is judged to be a clear and imminent threat to someone else—like your children—she may be involuntarily hospitalized. If the threat is not clear and imminent, but you feel that there is a possibility of danger, take immediate steps to have the children stay elsewhere, such as at a relative's house, until your partner has been stabilized.

Suicidality

Most people are aware of the risk of suicide during bipolar depression, but many don't realize there also is an increased prevalence of suicide among individuals with psychotic mania and mixed episodes (where manic and depressed symptoms appear concurrently).

Only a psychiatrist or psychologist who has received proper training can assess your partner for suicide risk, and I'll get into assessing suicidality and taking preventive measures in more depth in Chapter 9. But for now, know that you should **take any verbalization about suicide as legitimate and serious.** Do not assume that your mate is being manipulative or that the behavior is just a "cry for help." You are not in a position to judge your partner's intent—only a trained clinician can do this! You must have your mate evaluated for suicide risk by the doctor immediately if your partner expresses a desire to die. If the doctor judges that your loved one is an imminent risk to himself, your partner may be hospitalized involuntarily for a specified period of time in order to further assess the situation and protect your mate from self-inflicted harm.

> "I wish I was dead."
>
> "It would be better if I weren't here."
>
> "I want to die."
>
> "I'm going to kill myself."

Psychosis

Your partner may inadvertently put herself in harm's way because of actions she takes related to delusions or hallucinations. As I discussed in Chapter 4, antipsychotic medications usually are used to treat manic psychosis. However, at times you may have to deal with your

Talking to a Loved One Who Is Manic

Don't ...

- *Try to reason.* Mania is by its very nature an unreasonable condition.
- *Confront or corner* your partner. You need to deescalate, not escalate, the situation.
- *Blame* your partner for his or her current condition. Even if your mate is manic because of something he or she did or did not do, being accusatory will not help the situation.
- *Threaten* ("You do this or else"). This may propel your partner into behaving in the very way you're trying to avoid.
- *"Take the bait."* Don't respond to your partner's attempts to engage you in an argument or debate. Statements that begin with "You never ... " or "You don't ... " more often than not should be ignored.

Do ...

- *Listen and reflect* back what you hear your partner saying. For example, say, "I understand that you're feeling _____" or "I hear you saying that _____."
- Speak in a *calm and even* manner.
- *Ask* what you can do to help; don't "tell." For example, in response to your partner's sharing with you how angry he or she is feeling, you may say, "I understand that you're feeling angry. What can we do to make you feel less this way?"
- Use *gentle persuasion.* For instance, "I know that you reduced your medication recently (on your own). Maybe it would be a good idea if you went back to your usual dose?"

---

mate when she is having delusional beliefs or suffering from auditory, visual, tactile, or olfactory hallucinations.

Delusions

Delusions are false, unshakable beliefs that are acted on. Manic delusions frequently are grandiose or paranoid. Grandiose delusions can involve your partner's believing (and acting accordingly) that he is some very important figure from the present or past (a famous actor; a historical figure of great stature) or that he has some special power or ability (can read minds or fly). Paranoid delusions usually are persecutory in nature. Your mate may believe other people are talking about, watching, or following him, some kind of conspiratorial activity is taking place around him, or that he is in danger.

Let me say at the outset, **you cannot reason with someone who has a delusion.** By their very nature, delusions do not respond to logic—although untrue, those who have them firmly believe them; they are fixed or "cemented" in place. So you need to know that you will not be able to "talk" your mate out of his delusions.

A delusion is ...
 A faulty, fixed belief that a person acts on.
Delusional themes often are ...
 Grandiose or persecutory (paranoid).

You also don't want to support whatever false idea your mate has in mind. If you agree that someone is, for example, conspiring against your partner, you will escalate rather than attenuate the situation. So what do you do instead?

- *Be a good listener.* Hear what your partner has to say without criticizing, judging, or pointing out flaws in her logic.
- *Acknowledge that your partner is having distressing thoughts.* For instance, you might say, "I know that you believe that _____ is following you" or "I understand that you think you are under surveillance."
- *Be reassuring.* In a calm but firm manner, let your mate know that he has your support (without validating his distorted perception) by saying something nonspecific like "We'll do whatever we need to in order to keep you safe," "I'm always there for you," or "Whatever's wrong, we'll take care of it."

Hallucinations

During a hallucination, a person actually sees (visual), hears (auditory), feels (tactile), or smells (olfactory) something that, in fact, isn't there. Like delusions, the content of hallucinations often is grandiose or persecutory, although sometimes it's just, frankly, bizarre.

Raoul—*visual hallucination (persecutory):*

> "I looked up and I saw these huge monsters, like they were 8 feet tall and grotesque looking. They were running after the people in the street and killing them. There was blood everywhere. I ran as fast as I could to hide from them. I ran so fast that I fell onto the concrete in the street and put a gash in my head. But I didn't have time to deal with it. I just kept on running."

Jean—*tactile hallucination (bizarre):*

> "I could feel the worms coming out of every pore in my body. They are really hard to see, but if you look real close you can see them. I went to the hospital emergency room to get a doctor to look at them under the microscope, thinking he would give me something to get rid of them. I believed it was the worms that were making me sick, not bipolar disorder."

Betsy—*auditory hallucination (persecutory):*

> "The voice was a man's voice, no one I knew. He was telling me to kill myself, to climb onto the roof and jump off. The voice said I was evil and deserved to die. But I knew it was him that was evil, not me. I fought as hard as I could not to go up on the roof. It was one of the hardest things I've ever had to do."

Jared—*visual hallucination (grandiose):*

> "I looked in the mirror and I saw God. I mean the reflection that looked back at me was Jesus's. I thought, 'I'm God. I can do anything. I'm all-powerful.' With knowing who I was came a feeling of great excitement. Everything now was finally beginning to make sense. I wasn't 'crazy'; I had a destiny to fulfill!"

A hallucination is . . .
A perceptual experience in the absence of an identifiable stimulus.

Hallucinations may be . . .
Auditory—hearing voices that aren't there.
Visual—seeing an image that isn't there.
Tactile—feeling something that isn't there.
Olfactory—smelling something that isn't there.

Gwen—olfactory hallucination (persecutory):

> *"I was lying in my bed, and I could smell the distinct odor of gas. It was everywhere, all over the house. I woke my husband up, but he said he didn't smell anything. I knew it was there, and I was afraid the gas was poisonous and I would die. I wasn't sure whether my being gassed was an accident or someone wanted to hurt me. I just knew that I had to get out of there, and so I did."*

As you can imagine, hallucinations can be very frightening to those who have them. They also, as I'm sure you gathered from the examples above, can be dangerous, because of the actions people take based on their faulty perceptions. The best thing you can do to help your mate if he is having a hallucination (besides making absolutely sure that he

Manic (or Mixed) Emergencies

Type of emergency	What to do
Suicidal	Call your partner's psychiatrist. If you can't reach the doctor, and you think your partner is in imminent danger, take him to the hospital; if he refuses to go, call the police.
Aggressive/dangerous to you/others	If your partner is an imminent threat to you or others, immediately call the police.
Delusions, hallucinations	Call your partner's doctor. If you can't reach the doctor and the content of your partner's delusions or hallucinations make her an imminent danger to herself or someone else, take her to the hospital; if she refuses to go, call the police.
Extremely disruptive (for example, screaming in the middle of the street at 3:00 A.M., etc.)	Call your partner's doctor. If you can't reach the doctor, take him to the hospital. If the disruptive behavior poses an imminent threat to your partner or someone else, and he is unwilling to go to the hospital, call the police.
Unable to care for self	Call your partner's psychiatrist to schedule an emergency visit.

is taking the antipsychotic medicine the doctor prescribed, exactly *as* prescribed) is to provide a safe and reassuring environment. However, if the content of your mate's hallucination (or delusion) potentially poses a threat to his well-being (as, for instance, in Betsy's case) or is a danger to someone else, you have an emergency situation on your hands and you must immediately contact your partner's physician or, if you can't get through to the doctor right away, take your mate to the nearest emergency room. If your partner doesn't cooperate, you may have no choice other than to call the police, who are accustomed to dealing with situations of this sort.

The Behavioral Contract

A behavioral contract essentially is a signed agreement between you and your partner regarding preventive measures that will be put in place in the event your mate shows signs of becoming ill. When used for mania, the contract specifies what each of you will commit to doing when early warning signs of mania appear. It gives you something to refer to in the event that your partner denies getting ill, as so many people do when mania starts to take hold. I strongly advise that you put such a contract in place if your partner has a history of engaging in high-risk behaviors when hypomanic or manic.

The contract should be drawn up at a time when your mate is not in a mood episode—neither manic nor depressed. It specifies what each of you will do when you observe certain symptoms—the early warning signs you wrote down on page 206—to prevent your mate from getting worse and what safeguards will be instituted to protect your partner and her loved ones. Actions you'll each take to prevent your mate's mania from worsening can include items from the early intervention plan on pages 209–211, as well as any other measure whose goal is to increase mood stability (see Chapter 7 for detailed information on a variety of such measures).

If and when your partner shows early warning signs, you should produce the document and review it together, reminding your mate that he agreed to take these precautions in the event of a mood shift like the one that is occurring now, to protect him and other family members.

Behavioral Contract for Mania

List your partner's typical early warning signs of hypomania or mania (transfer what you wrote on page 206 to the following spaces):

_____

_____

_____

_____

List what actions your mate will take when the symptoms specified above first appear (for example, calling the psychiatrist, increasing the frequency of therapy sessions, avoiding alcohol, going to bed at a regular hour, telling spouse or doctor if having suicidal thoughts, turning over the car keys, avoiding risky sexual situations, surrendering the charge cards, taking medication in front of spouse, etc.):

_____

_____

_____

_____

List what actions you will take when the symptoms specified above first appear (for example, removing alcohol from the home; shouldering more of the responsibilities at home; checking in with your partner on a regular basis; having a hospital in place, just in case; having the children stay with a relative; etc.):

_____

_____

_____

_____

What about My Feelings?

You may, as many of my patients' partners report, experience a range of intense—often negative—emotions when going through a period of mania with your mate. What can you do about these feelings to ensure they don't sap your strength and threaten your own health?

Angry

"I'm getting mad when he gets angry, which only compounds the problem."

Make sure you aren't "taking the bait" (see the sidebar on page 221)—that you aren't responding to your partner's verbal attacks in a similar manner. If you find you just can't seem to avoid doing this, consider taking some time away from the situation. Can you leave your partner alone for an afternoon or evening? If not, is there someone you trust whom you can ask to be a stand-in just for a few hours? (And make sure you use that time away to do something special that's just for you—see Chapter 10 for some suggestions.)

Guilty

"It's wrong that I'm feeling this way. She's sick; it's not her fault."

You feel guilty about the negative emotions you're having in response to your mate. But please know that the way you are feeling (angry, scared, etc.)—regardless of which particular emotion it is—is completely understandable and normal. I wouldn't have included it here if it weren't!

If you are feeling bad about your reactions, you may benefit from talking with others who are in a situation similar to yours, by seeking out a support group (in person or via the Internet). Knowing that you are not alone in how you are feeling can help a great deal.

Sad

"I'm feeling so sad—not like my normal self."

When your partner is manic, you are, in a very real way, experiencing a loss, and losses bring with them feelings of sadness. The person you know is absent, and your relationship, for lack of a better term, is "temporarily suspended" or "on hold," since you really can't have a meaningful partnership with someone who is manic.

If your sadness is very intense and pervasive, you may actually be in a depression—in which case you will benefit from much of what's included in Chapter 9. Also consider getting some help from a professional, which I'll talk about in Chapter 10.

Scared

"I'm frightened by the way my partner is acting."

Are you feeling scared because your partner is psychotic, suicidal, physically expressing intense rage, or involved in dangerous activities? If your answer is "yes" to any of these, you have good reason to feel afraid. In all likelihood it means that your mate's illness has progressed to the point that he needs to be in a hospital. Immediately contact your mate's doctor. If you can't reach your partner's physician and you feel there is some imminent danger or threat present, take your mate to the nearest emergency room or, if necessary, contact the police.

Hurt

"My spouse says very hurtful things to me."

I know that when your partner is yelling hurtful comments it can be hard to remember that this is the illness talking, not the person you love. At a time like this, it's important to remember that manic episodes are just that—episodes; in other words, *they pass.* Your mate is not going to be like this forever and, in all likelihood, she will return pretty much to how she was before the mania occurred. Try to keep that picture of your spouse in your mind during this very trying period. In fact, it actually may be helpful to jot down some characteristics of your mate—ones that reflect her "true self," not the illness, but rather the person you love.

Lonely

"When he's manic, I really feel alone. It's like I've lost my best friend."

Although it may not be easy to do, it's very important to maintain your other close relationships during this difficult time. Connecting with friends and relatives will make you feel less socially isolated and emotionally alone. If you can't do it in person, then at least pick up the telephone and call them. And, again, as I said earlier, consider a support group—it's not only a safe place to express your feelings but also an opportunity to form meaningful connections with other people.

When You Feel You Can't Go On

Manic behavior definitely takes a toll on well partners, so much so that during episodes people may find themselves questioning whether they want to remain committed to their partners. Although in the midst of an episode you may seriously contemplate "calling it quits," before you further entertain this option take some time to honestly examine your relationship by asking yourself the following questions:

- How much of the time is my mate in an episode? Does the amount of "ill time" exceed the amount of "well time"? If "yes," are there other avenues (of treatment) that could be explored that might increase the length of my mate's well periods?
- Looking at the "well periods," how content or happy am I in my relationship? Is there anything I could do, alone or together with my partner, to improve our relationship?
- Would the quality of my life be enhanced by no longer having my partner in it? If "yes," how? Are there ways to achieve this without leaving the relationship?
- What would I miss about my relationship if it were to end?
- What feasibility issues (finances, children) would I have to deal with if my spouse and I were to separate?

I think that when you look at the answers to the preceding questions you'll find, despite the very real difficulties that come with having a relationship with a bipolar individual, that there are plenty of reasons why you've remained with your partner. However, if, on the other hand, you find that the weight of the evidence suggests you need to seriously consider the possibility of terminating your relationship, see Chapter 10 for help in dealing with this very difficult decision.

Anxious

"I'm feeling really uptight."

Are you surprised that you feel this way? If you are, you shouldn't be. You're going through an incredibly stressful time living with someone who is completely unpredictable, possibly even a danger to herself or someone else in your family.

As best you can, try to take some time to participate in activities that will reduce your overall level of tension, such as some form of exercise, physical activities around the home, or playing a sport. Relaxation techniques, yoga, and/or meditation also can be extremely helpful (see Resources).

Exhausted

"I've been completely worn down by dealing with his manic behavior."

Even though your partner is ill, it's important that you have some time for yourself away from your mate. If you feel guilty at the prospect of spending time apart, consider that keeping a constant "vigil" is not going to do you or your mate any good—you will get run down and ultimately be of less help to your partner.

If, however, your mate's condition indicates that he should not be left alone, consider having someone you trust (like another family member or a really close friend) fill in for you, even if only for a few hours. This will give you the break you need and deserve.

Hopeless

"I feel like we're on a roller coaster ride that's never going to end."

Maybe this is a good time to take a step back and look at your partner's treatment plan. Consider having a talk with your partner's doctor about other treatment options or even consulting another doctor to get a second opinion. And remember that new treatments for bipolar disorder are being developed all the time—there is never a reason to give up hope!

What Do I Tell Other People?

Should you disclose information about your partner's current condition? If "yes," to whom should you disclose, and how much should you reveal? These are questions you undoubtedly will have to deal with in the event your partner has a full-blown manic episode.

Friends and Relatives

Deciding which friends and relatives to tell about your partner's episode depends on a number of factors:

- Is there some advantage to a particular individual's knowing about your mate's current condition? For example, could he be helping you out in some way while your partner is not well?
- Is the individual in close geographical proximity? In other words, what is the feasibility of keeping information from this person?
- Does your partner have regularly scheduled events together with this person, like dinner together every Sunday or bridge every Thursday, so that your mate's absence would require an explanation?
- How close is your partner to this friend/relative? Is she someone your partner would want to know what was going on?
- Is this someone you and your mate can trust with delicate information of this sort? Or is the person someone who would in some way use the information against your partner? Does this individual have anything to gain from your family's misfortune?
- Has your partner already exhibited unusual behavior in front of this individual, so that an explanation really is called for?

Once you determine the person(s) you need to say something to, you'll have to consider what exactly you want to say. In other words, how much do you want to share?

In some cases, it may be sufficient to say something vague, like "_____ has been under the weather" or "_____ hasn't been feeling well," implying (although not directly stating) that the problem is physical in nature. However, if the friend or relative already knows that your spouse has bipolar disorder, it may be easiest (and, obviously, the most honest approach) to say that your partner has had a recurrence of the illness. It's really not necessary to specify that it's mania (as opposed to depression), unless you need to, for some reason, get into the details of the current situation with the individual (for instance, if your spouse is trying to talk this person's partner into going to Las Vegas for a weekend of gambling).

Employers

Deciding what to tell an employer can be trickier than determining what to share with a friend or relative. Obviously, your mate's livelihood is at stake here, and you want to make sure you don't do anything to risk that.

The first thing you want to assess—if you can—is approximately how long you think your partner will be away from work. I know, of course, that you can't predict the future (none of us can), but on the basis of your mate's history you may be able to make a rough estimate of how long it will be before he can resume work. For example, if your mate's acute manic episodes tend to be fairly short (days or a couple of weeks) and he typically returns quickly to his former level of functioning (no lingering residual symptoms or at least none that would interfere with his performance in any major way), you may want to consider the option of using sick time that's been accrued. Some people use personal or vacation time instead, but whether it's possible to take this time on very little advance notice depends on how your partner's employment contract is structured.

If you think your partner may be out for an extended period of time—many weeks or even months—you may have to consider the possibility of an unpaid leave of absence (for personal or medical reasons) or, if she has a disability policy as a benefit of her employment, applying for short- or long-term disability benefits.

Sometimes absences with certain employers require documentation, which means your partner will probably have to have a form filled out by his doctor (or have the doctor write a letter) specifying the nature of the infirmity. Although it, obviously, will be clear from such documentation that the problem is psychiatric, psychiatrists often are pretty adroit at keeping comments fairly general, so that your mate's employer won't know for sure what the exact condition is. I also want to point out that in the case of a prolonged absence you probably will be dealing with someone from the human resources (HR) department (provided your spouse's place of employment has one), not your mate's actual employer. HR people, as they are often referred to, typically have a lot of experience dealing with delicate situations of this sort. But keep in mind that their primary loyalty is to their employer, the person who signs their paychecks, not to you.

You also need to know that your partner, if disabled by her bipolar disorder, has certain rights under the law through the Americans with Disabilities Act, which requires employers to make reasonable accommodations for employees who have disabilities (including psychiatric). Of course, an employer must be aware of a person's illness to make any accommodations. Accommodations may include, for example, restricting traveling between different time zones, working regular day or evening shifts (rather than variable shifts), part-time rather than full-time work, having office or cubicle placement where there is less noise or fewer disruptions, being allowed to leave work for doctor's appointments (with an opportunity to make up the missed hours), being allowed to leave work at lunchtime to "destress" (exercise, use relaxation techniques, etc.).

Coworkers

What you decide to tell coworkers will depend to a large extent on two factors: (1) what is revealed to your mate's employer and (2) how close your partner is to a particular coworker. Obviously, if you are leading your partner's employer to believe the problem is purely physical, you need to carefully consider the potential consequences of giving other individuals in the same work environment conflicting information. It may be that in only a few—or, alternatively, in no—cases can you be confident that taking people into your confidence won't backfire and become "the latest news," to be shared indiscriminately around the building's water fountain. Remember, above all else you want to protect your mate's future in this job. Therefore, as a general rule of thumb, if you are in doubt about revealing "the truth," you probably are better off not doing so.

In this chapter you've learned how to identify your partner's early warning signs of mania and what actions to take when they occur. I've also discussed strategies for dealing with full-blown manic episodes—those that will help your mate, as well as ones that will make it easier for you to cope. Now let's turn our attention to the other end of the pendulum—depression.

Strategies for Dealing with the Downs Together

9

Brenner: *What are you still doing in bed?*

Robin: *I'm really depressed. I couldn't go in to work today.*

Brenner: *But your students are counting on you. They need you.*

Robin: *They can get along without me. In fact, everyone probably would be better off without me.*

Brenner: *That's your depression talking.*

Robin: *I'm a failure. My life has been completely meaningless.*

Brenner: *I don't know how you can say that. What about your career? Do you think that everyone can be a college professor?*

Robin: *Maybe I just faked my way through. I'm not that smart.*

Brenner: *You faked your way through 4 years of college, 4 years of graduate school, and then were able to pull the wool over the eyes of the math department's administration and your colleagues?*

Robin: *Uh, I guess that's a little far-fetched.*

Brenner: *Yes, very far-fetched.*

Robin: *But I'm feeling so stupid now. It's like there's cotton in my brain.*

Brenner: *You've been through this enough to know that it's the depression and that your thinking will improve as your mood gets better. And the way to get your mood better is to follow your normal routine. Staying home from work is not going to help you.*

Robin: *I know you're right, but it feels so hard to move.*

Brenner: *I know it's hard, but why don't you try to get dressed and then see how you feel?*

Robin: *Okay, I'll try. Maybe if I can get it together, I could still make it in for my afternoon class.*

Unlike experiencing mania and hypomania, which can be enjoyable, even intoxicating, nobody gets pleasure from being depressed. Depression is an excruciatingly painful experience that, to those afflicted, can seem insurmountable and without end.

But like mania, depression also damages people's lives—it just goes about it in a more insidious, less blatant, way. Depressed people slowly withdraw from the world, leaving behind their jobs, families, friends, and interests. They become very self-absorbed. By saying that, I don't mean egotistical. What I mean, rather, is that depression leads people to become *self-focused.* This is a critical distinction to understand, because if you haven't experienced depression yourself you might misinterpret depressed people's behavior as being self-indulgent or trying to manipulate others into paying attention to and taking care of them. And that's not the case at all.

Depressed people are incapable of the reciprocity that's crucial to maintaining relationships. Absorbed in their own pain, they can't give and also, in the true sense of the word, can't receive. As a result, well partners often suffer along with their loved ones—not only feeling bad for their ill mates, for what they are going through, but also experiencing the (temporary) loss of their primary relationships, often having feelings of isolation and sadness themselves.

Because depression is so devastating—both for your partner and for you—a good part of this chapter focuses on early identification and intervention. Knowing your partner's early warning signs of depression will enable the two of you to use early intervention methods that can turn things around before they worsen. However, in the event that your mate's depression progresses and becomes severe, I offer strategies you can use to help both of you get through it.

Identifying Early Warning Signs of Depression

Just like for mania, people have their own characteristic behaviors that suggest they are headed for a depression. I know that for me, feeling very tired despite adequate sleep, having a pessimistic outlook, and talking less are early warning signs that a down period is on its way. But as you can see in the list on the next page, many different behaviors can suggest the onset of a depressive episode.

When you look at the list, try to identify the early warning signs of depression that your partner has. I've also left room for you to fill in any behaviors that aren't included but that apply to your significant other. Once you've pinpointed your mate's early warning signs, fill them in on the form on page 239.

You may want to do this exercise along with your partner to get his input, especially if your mate is good at self-observation. Just make sure you complete the questionnaire at a time when your partner is not depressed, because depression can color one's perception of past events (as well as the present and future). And if the two of you don't agree on some of the early warning signs, don't get into an argument over it. Just agree to disagree and then consider going with the indicators you can agree on.

Remember that, in identifying early warning signs of depression, you want to make sure the behavior differs in some way—such as in frequency, duration, or intensity—from your partner's usual state. Let's say your loved one is, in general, "a crier," but when she begins to get depressed she is tearful *more often* than usual. Or your mate's busy schedule typically makes him feel tired at times, but when headed for a low period he complains of being fatigued virtually *all the time* or to the point of extreme exhaustion.

It's also important to keep in mind that early warning signs generally cluster together during the same time period; individually, they

Early Warning Signs of Depression

Circle all of the items that apply to your mate. Remember, for an item to count as a warning sign, it must represent a change from your partner's usual behavior during periods of normal mood.

Crying

Quiet or less talkative

Sleeping in

Taking "sick days" from work

Little enthusiasm for doing things

Taking naps during the day

Drinking more

Complaining of being bored

Tired

Eating less

Complaining that food doesn't taste as good or the same

Complaining of not feeling good in general or of specific physical problems (aches or pains)

Not as "sharp" as usual

Preoccupied

Complaining of being tired a lot

Uninterested or less interested in being with other people

Eating more

Less interested in sex

Indecisive

Dwelling or focusing on the negative

Less attentive to personal grooming

Not answering the phone

Wanting to be alone

Other behaviors: _____

_____

_____

_____

_____

_____

My Partner's Early Warning Signs of Depression

List at least three changes that appear together (during the same period of time) at the very beginning of your partner's depressive episodes.

Early Warning Sign #1:

_____

_____

Early Warning Sign #2:

_____

_____

Early Warning Sign #3:

_____

_____

Early Warning Sign #4:

_____

_____

Early Warning Sign #5:

_____

_____

may have no real significance. For example, a somewhat decreased appetite in and of itself may not be a cause for concern, but when accompanied by increased alcohol intake and trouble sleeping, *together* these symptoms may alert you to the possibility that a mood problem is brewing.

Greg knows his wife, Virginia, is headed for a depression when he sees these signs: sleeping 1 or 2 hours more a night, complaining of feeling tired a lot, eating more sweets than usual, not making social plans, and less interested in sex.

How can Greg share what he's worried about with his wife without her feeling bad about it and possibly becoming even more depressed? He needs to show sensitivity and compassion in the way he approaches the topic, realizing that, in her current mood state, Virginia is likely to take whatever he says very much to heart.

Greg: Honey, I'm worried about how you've been feeling lately. You just don't seem like yourself.

Virginia: I didn't want you to know that I was beginning to slip. Now I feel even worse, knowing that you see what's happening. I don't want to do this to you again. I don't want to make your life miserable.

Greg: Listen, you have an illness that you didn't choose to have. And you're not in a depression now anyway. You're just showing some early signs that we should be grateful we noticed. Because this means we can do something about it now and turn things around so you don't have to have another bad period again.

Virginia: I don't know how to turn things around. I just feel like I'm sinking deeper.

Greg: That's why we should contact your doctor. Let him know what's going on so he can adjust your medication.

Virginia: I don't want the doctor to know I'm not feeling well. I'm embarrassed that I get like this. I don't want anyone to know.

Greg: You don't need to be embarrassed in front of your own doctor. He understands bipolar disorder—he sees people with it all the time. He's not going to blame you or think less of you for having a mood shift.

Virginia: I don't care. I'm not calling him. I can't face telling him.

Greg: Well, what if I give him a call? He can tell me what he thinks we should do. You don't have to get on the phone if you don't want to. I promise.

Virginia: Okay, just as long as I don't have to speak to him.

As it ended up, after Greg spoke to the doctor for a few minutes Virginia did get on the phone. Having Greg "pave the road" made it easier for her to talk to the doctor and share what was going on with her.

But what if Virginia had continued to give Greg a hard time about contacting the doctor? By waiting a bit and trying again Greg might have gotten through to his wife.

Sometimes the well partner will see the early warning signs of depression but the mate is reluctant to accept that it's true. This was the case with Rebecca and Roger:

Rebecca: Roger, when is your next appointment with your psychiatrist?

Roger: Next month. Why are you asking?

Rebecca: Because I've noticed some things—nothing major, but enough that I think you need to check in with her.

Roger: What are you talking about? I'm fine.

Rebecca: Well, you've been drinking more than usual and going to sleep really early.

Roger: I've had a lot of stress at work lately. You know that business has been bad the last few months.

Rebecca: I know, but drinking and sleeping a lot are signs that you may be beginning to get depressed. It's understandable, with business being so off, but still, I think we need to pay attention to it.

Roger: I can't deal with getting depressed again.

Rebecca: But if you do something about it now, there's a good chance it won't get to that point. Which is why I wanted to know when you're scheduled to see the doctor.

Roger: Do you think it's so bad that it can't wait till next month?

Rebecca: Not necessarily, but why take the chance? I think you should move it up, just to be on the safe side.

Roger: Maybe you're right. I guess I have nothing to lose.

The Early Intervention Plan

As the preceding examples highlighted, letting the other members of the treatment team—your partner's doctors—know about your mate's mood shift is a very important step in helping to ensure that a minor depression doesn't become more severe. However, as you'll see below, there also are a number of other concrete measures your mate or the two of you can take to help turn things around:

1. *Encourage your mate to set small goals and break them down into feasible steps.* Setting and meeting goals enhances self-esteem and elevates mood. However, a goal shouldn't be too large, or it will have the reverse (undesired) effect. For example, if the house needs to be straightened up but it seems like an overwhelming task to your partner, suggest that she break the job down, room by room, and start with the room that will be easiest to get in order. Or, if the idea of cleaning one entire room seems like too large a step, break that down even further, by tackling just one component of the job, like hanging up clothes or dusting the furniture.

2. *Help your partner stay physically active.* When becoming depressed, people frequently decrease their level of physical activity. Staying active is more important now than ever. Has your mate stopped going to the gym? Has he decreased his regular tennis games from twice to once a week? Is there a way you can encourage him to return to his previous activity schedule? For example, if he's complaining that he can't manage his daily run in the mornings because he's tired, could you help out by getting up with him and making the coffee (providing him with the caffeine "boost" he needs to get going)? Are there physical activities that the two of you might take on together?

3. *Help your partner include pleasant events in each day.* Everyone needs activities and events that make him or her feel good. Is your mate so bogged down in doing the necessary stuff—work, caring for the kids, doing chores—that there really doesn't seem to be time for pleasure or fun? Could you help out to make some room in her busy schedule, maybe watching the kids for an hour in the evening so she can enjoy a bath or read a good book? Doing the laundry on Saturday while she goes for a run with a friend? Or getting someone else to help out—like getting a babysitter for Sunday afternoon so the two of you can go to the movies? Also keep in mind the little things

you could do to brighten her day—like bringing home a small bouquet of flowers or stopping at the store to pick up her favorite flavor of ice cream.

4. *Suggest that your mate increase exposure to light.* As you know from Chapter 4, exposure to light helps to elevate mood. Has your partner been getting enough outdoor time? Are there activities (perhaps physical ones—that way your mate will be accomplishing two of the items on this list at once) that the two of you could do together outside the house? Taking a walk, playing tennis, cross-country skiing? Or just sitting in the backyard listening to music, reading, or talking?

5. *Assist your loved one in maintaining contact with family and friends.* When people are beginning to get depressed, they frequently start to isolate from others. Make an effort to keep to your normal social calendar. If Sunday dinner is always with your partner's parents, continue the tradition. If your mate has a standing appointment to play cards with "the guys" on Tuesdays, encourage him to keep it, even if he's not as enthusiastic about it as usual.

6. *Persuade your partner to postpone making major life decisions.* Since depression impairs judgment, now definitely isn't a good time to make plans that will have a major impact on your lives. You can actually say something of this sort to your partner: "I've read that people should put off making major life decisions when depressed. How about we put this decision on hold until you're feeling better?" Or consider using yourself as the scapegoat, saying something like "I've got so much on my mind right now. Can we wait on this until things lighten up for me?"

7. *Try to adhere as closely as possible to a normal routine.* You already know from Chapter 7 the importance of having a regular routine for mood stability. Has there recently been a change in the usual routine, one that's affecting your mate? Or, when you think back, have you and your mate gotten a bit "loose" lately about keeping to your daily schedule? Have you been eating meals catch-as-catch-can? Going to bed whenever the mood strikes? Do your best to get back on your usual routine—with set times for meals and sleep.

8. *If you can identify a trigger situation, take steps to eliminate it or lessen its impact.* In Chapter 7 you identified your mate's triggers for depression. Have any of these situations occurred recently (or are any present now)? If so, is the circumstance something that can be removed or reversed so that it no longer has an impact on your mate?

Or are there steps you can take to minimize the effect the trigger is having? For example, if your family recently lost a pet, maybe it would help to bring a new puppy/kitten into the home. If the two of you haven't been spending as much quality time together, perhaps planning a vacation (if feasible) would help to rekindle the relationship. Could the trigger be hormonal in nature and a visit to the gynecologist or endocrinologist be of help?

9. *Keep in close contact with your mate.* Checking in on a regular basis, for example, at three o'clock every afternoon, lets your mate know that you are thinking of him and that you care and are there. It's also a way to monitor any further mood fluctuations. Don't, though, check in too often (telephone calls numerous times a day) or your mate might begin to worry that he is even worse than he thought.

10. *Make sure all members of the treatment team are aware of the current situation.* Sharing early warning signs with your partner's medical doctor allows the physician to intervene early—to make adjustments in medication that can help ward off another mood episode. And if your mate is in therapy, she may want to ask about the possibility of increasing the frequency of the sessions, just until she is feeling more level again.

What If There's No Time for the Early Intervention Plan?

Sometimes—particularly when it's immediately following a manic or hypomanic episode—a major depression will appear without early warning signs. It actually is like falling off the edge of a cliff. One minute your mate's mood is elevated, and then, literally without warning, it takes a nosedive. This is the pattern that I have tended to experience throughout my illness.

Thankfully, I haven't had a major depressive episode in a long time, but that doesn't mean I don't remember what it felt like. I recall my first episode, feeling beyond sad—completely numb and empty, like I had experienced a tremendous loss (like you might expect from losing a spouse). Although numb, I felt, paradoxically, emotional pain that was almost unbearable. Each day of living was torture, and each one of the days felt like an eternity. Sleep was my only refuge, but given my sleep difficulties, it was hard to come by. I got no pleasure from anything, including food, which tasted like cardboard and seemed to catch in my throat. Most of the time I spent immobilized in what used to be my favorite chair but had then turned into my prison. When I did venture out, it seemed like everywhere I turned there were smiling faces and laughter, which only deepened my sense of despair and confirmed my perception that I was different from other people, making me feel even more alone.

If this is something like the situation you and your partner find yourself in, one of you (your partner may be too incapacitated to do this on his own) will need to contact your mate's physician. Your mate's psychiatrist will probably want to see your partner right away. At that appointment the doctor will evaluate the severity of your spouse's depression and determine two things: (1) whether your partner needs to be in a hospital (see the sidebar on page 249 for the benefits of psychiatric hospitalization) and (2) whether any adjustments need to be made in the current medication schedule.

If your partner is not currently maintained on an antidepressant, the doctor may consider adding one under certain circumstances. As explained in Chapter 4, antidepressants are generally prescribed for bipolar depression only in conjunction with a mood stabilizer. Even then, according to recent guidelines, they should be used only for severe bipolar depression or where mood stabilizers alone have failed to be effective.

It's also important to keep in mind that individuals vary considerably in their idiosyncratic responses to antidepressants. Unfortunately, at this time there is no fail-proof way to predict which particular drug will have a significant antidepressant effect for your loved one. As a result, the doctor may have to go through several trials of different antidepressants to arrive at the one that works for your partner. Try to be patient and optimistic.

In addition to getting the medication component in place for your mate, there are a number of things the two of you should pay attention to—what I refer to as the "basics" in fighting a severe depression. Encourage your partner to:

- *Attend to personal grooming and get dressed* (out of the robe, pajamas, etc.) each day, even if your partner is not going to be leaving the house.
- *Stay out of bed*, except for normal sleep hours. If your mate

feels immobilized by depression, he can sit somewhere else (for example, outside on the patio, if weather permits, would be a good option), but should steer clear of the bed.

- *Answer the telephone*, even though your loved one might not feel like talking. It's important for your mate not to completely socially isolate herself.
- *Move around*, even though your partner may complain of having no energy. Taking a short walk or even going up and down the stairs repeatedly helps by maintaining at least a minimal level of physical activity.
- *Keep curtains, blinds, etc., open* to let the sunlight in. As you know, bright light has an antidepressant effect, so make sure it's streaming into your home. Also keep the house filled with artificial light at night.
- *Eat regular meals*, even if your mate is not hungry, because low blood sugar will worsen his mood. If your partner finds he is having difficulty forcing himself to eat, try foods that "go down easy," like soup, pasta, applesauce, ice cream, and/or planning smaller, more frequent mini-meals.
- *Schedule at least one activity each day* so your partner has some feeling of accomplishment. The activity might be a household chore (doing the wash, cleaning the kitchen), running an errand (going to the supermarket, dry cleaner, drugstore), or spending time on a work-related task that can be performed at home.
- *Indulge in a bit of pampering.* Your loved one should do little things that make her feel better (even if only the smallest bit), such as getting a manicure, eating a chocolate bar, watching a favorite TV program, taking a bubble bath, reading a good book or magazine.
- *Watch out for depressive "self-talk."* Replace negative thoughts with more positive alternatives. For example, if your mate thinks/says, "I'll never get better," he can replace it with, or you can respond with, "Depression always passes." If your spouse spends long periods of time silently dwelling on the negatives, encourage him to cut them short by scheduling worry time, as discussed in Chapter 7.
- *Adhere to the treatment plan.* Take all medications—including any new ones—exactly as prescribed by the doctor. Keep all scheduled medication and therapy appointments—do not can-

Talking to a Loved One Who Is Depressed

Don't . . .

- *Minimize the problem.* For example, don't say, "It can't be that bad" or "You'll feel better when you see this beautiful day!"
- *Ask for answers.* Not only are questions like "Why are you depressed?" a waste of time, but not having an answer will make your partner feel worse.
- *Use "tough love."* For example, don't say, "Buck up," "Snap out of it," or "Pull yourself up by your bootstraps."
- *Try to talk or reason your partner out of being depressed.* Statements like "But you've got everything going for you" or "There are a lot of people worse off than you" are not helpful. On the other hand, pointing out cognitive distortions and faulty logic, in a gentle, nonconfrontational way (see the example at the beginning of this chapter), can help your partner.
- *Criticize* your mate, even if you consider it constructive criticism. Your spouse feels bad enough about herself without your adding to the mix.

Do . . .

- *Listen, comfort, and reassure.* Let your partner do the talking and make sure he knows you hear what he is saying. Say things like "We'll get through this together" and "I love you and I'm here for you." Also, reassure your partner that he is not "a burden," that he is ill and you are helping just like he would do for you.
- *Look for opportunities to praise your partner.* Everyone likes to hear compliments and receive praise, but depressed people are especially in need of positive attention. Even praise for the small things will help, like saying "Your hair looks really pretty today," "That wax job you did on the car looks terrific," or "Dinner tonight was great."
- *Let your partner know that there is "light at the end of the tunnel."* Your partner needs to be reminded, possibly quite frequently, that she won't feel this way forever, that depressions are time-limited—they pass. For example, you might say, "You've been through this before, and you know it will end; it won't be like this forever" or "We just need to wait for the medicine to work, and then you'll begin to feel better."
- *Be a cheerleader.* Encourage your partner to take steps to fight the depression, saying things like "I know you can do it" or "Why don't you give it a try?" Try to stay as upbeat and positive as possible.

cel or postpone visits because of not feeling up to it or because of being too depressed.

Years ago, to help get me moving during a very lethargic depression, my husband literally held my arm and walked me up and down the hall of our single-story home, encouraging me every step of the way. If that's what you need to do to help your mate stay mobile during a severe depression, then by all means do it.

Cara found the only thing that made her feel at all better during her depression was for her husband to "cuddle" with her in bed. While I typically do not recommend spending time in bed other than to sleep when one is depressed, for Cara spending 30 minutes or so embracing and snuggling with her spouse apparently gave her the emotional fortitude to face the day.

What to Watch Out For

As I mentioned earlier, despite all of your efforts, and the efforts of the doctors who are prescribing medication and providing therapy, your partner's depression might continue to worsen and/or go on so long that further measures need to be considered, such as ECT (see Chapter 4) or psychiatric hospitalization (see the sidebar below).

How do you know if your loved one's illness has progressed to this point? If your mate's doctor has tried numerous combinations of medications for her over many months but she continues to have severe depressive symptoms and can't function in her usual role (for example, at home, or at school or work), and/or potentially poses some type of harm to herself (for example, because of substance abuse, suicidal thoughts/urges, or psychotic behavior), it's time to talk to your partner's psychiatrist about other medical options.

Alcohol Abuse

I can't emphasize strongly enough that *alcohol and depression are a disastrous, and even potentially lethal, combination.* As I've said numerous times previously in this book, alcohol worsens the severity and increases the length of depressive episodes and dramatically increases the risk of suicide.

Psychiatric Hospitalization: What Are the Benefits?

- Provides *protection* from accidental or intentional self-harm or neglect for suicidal, substance-abusing, or psychotic individuals and/or those who do not demonstrate basic self-care (eating, sleeping, showering, etc.)
- Provides a set, daily *routine* with scheduled events (mealtimes, bedtime, etc.) and activities (exercise, therapy, etc.)
- Promotes *interaction* with staff and other patients
- Can help to establish or firm up the *diagnosis*
- Includes frequent—often daily—*therapeutic contact* with mental health practitioners (individual therapy, group therapy, medication management sessions)
- Offers a controlled and safe environment in which to withdraw from and/or add new *medication*

If your loved one is drinking alcohol, you need to do everything you can to motivate him to stop. Follow the suggestions I gave in Chapter 7, like keeping your home "dry" and eliminating activities that revolve around alcohol.

Suicidality

> *"Everything felt hopeless. I was certain that I was never going to get better, that the pain was never going to go away. I couldn't live like that anymore. So I started cutting back on my lithium and refilled my prescriptions early so I'd accumulate a lot. I'd heard that if you took enough of it, it would kill you. Fortunately my husband found out before it was too late."*

> *"I drive over the same bridge every day on the way to and from work. Lately, I can't get out of my mind the image of my running the car through the railing and over the side of the bridge, plummeting into the water below. I think, 'Now it will all be over. I won't have to suffer anymore.' But I don't know if I'll really go through with it."*

"It would be so easy. I have a gun. All I have to do is pull the trigger. Then all of my problems would be solved. I wouldn't have to worry about anything anymore. I'd finally be at peace."

The most catastrophic potential consequence of having a depression is, of course, taking one's own life. People usually are motivated to attempt suicide either because their emotional pain seems intolerable and endless or because they feel like they are facing an insurmountable obstacle (or obstacles).

While it would be reasonable to assume that your partner is at greatest risk for attempting suicide when most depressed, people who experience very severe depressions actually are most likely to attempt suicide when their depressions are just beginning to lift (it's thought that severely depressed people may be too incapacitated to actually take the actions that would be necessary to end their lives). Keep in mind, though, that these are findings based on averages of groups of individuals and therefore may not apply to your partner. You should never ignore "suicide red flags" regardless of the phase of depression your mate currently is going through.

Certain thoughts and behaviors should alert you to the possibility that your mate is considering self-harm:

- Seems *preoccupied with death and dying.* For example, your partner is talking about what it's like to be dead or is reading a book on dying or a "how to" guide to taking one's life.
- Makes *disturbing statements*, like:
  "I want to be dead."
  "I want to be with [someone who is already dead]."
  "I don't want to wake up tomorrow."
  "I'm going to kill myself."
- Seems to be *getting his affairs in order*, such as making changes to his will, giving you a list of bank accounts, putting all the assets in your name, taking out a life insurance policy.
- *Behaving secretively or in a suspicious manner.* Your partner seems to be keeping something from you—gets off the phone or shuts off the computer in a hurry when you enter the room or is suddenly unavailable at an unusual time or for a prolonged period of time.
- *Appears to be securing the means to commit self-harm*, such as

purchasing a firearm or "stockpiling" (amassing large quantities of a drug by reducing the dose for a period of time or refilling prescriptions prematurely) medication.

Although there are factors associated with increased risk, research has shown that it is not possible to accurately predict whether or when an individual will attempt to take his or her own life. That's why it's critical to pay attention to *any indication* that your loved one is thinking or behaving in a way that suggests she may be considering self-harm.

If you think your mate is at risk, you or your mate must call your partner's doctor(s) immediately to schedule an emergency appointment. When you call the doctor's office, make sure you say you need an *emergency* appointment, which should be scheduled the same day (unless you are calling in the evening or on the weekend—if you call after hours or at another time when the doctor is unavailable, you may be instructed to take your partner to the emergency room of the nearest hospital or to a psychiatric hospital where the doctor has staff privileges). ***Do not, under any circumstances, leave your partner alone*** while the two of you are waiting for the appointment, even if it's just for a few hours.

During the visit your partner's risk of suicide will be assessed

---

What the Doctor Looks for in Assessing Suicide Risk

- Feelings of *hopelessness*
- *Recent* suicidal statements
- *Frequent* suicidal statements
- A *plan* for administering self-harm
- The *intent* to do self-harm
- *Past suicide attempts*
- *Suicide in the family tree*
- Serious *medical illness or physical pain*
- Recent *psychiatric hospitalization*

What You Can Do to Keep Your Partner Safe

- Call the doctor immediately. If you can't reach the doctor and you feel the situation is urgent, take your mate to the emergency room. If he resists, call the police.
- Remove all alcohol from the home.
- Get rid of any weapons in the home.
- Take charge of your mate's medication. Make sure she is not in possession of large quantities of any psychiatric drug.
- Stay in close physical proximity to your mate. If you feel the situation is critical, do not even let your partner out of eyesight.
- Have in place a contract for suicide prevention (see page 254) that specifies what each of you will do in the event your mate is suicidal.

---

thoroughly, and if the doctor thinks your mate is at risk, she will work with you to develop and implement a plan to keep your partner safe. The plan may include a psychiatric hospitalization that, in addition to protecting your loved one, has other benefits for depression (see the sidebar on page 249). Even if your mate is opposed to the idea of a hospitalization, your partner can be held against his will ("involuntary hospitalization" or "involuntary commitment") if his judgment is considered impaired (meaning he can't determine whether treatment would be in his best interest) and he is deemed an *imminent danger to himself* or someone else. The specific procedure for involuntarily committing someone to a psychiatric hospital varies from state to state and may be enacted differently from community to community within a given state, but in all cases there are strict rules and safeguards to prevent abuses from occurring.

Psychosis

Although people don't usually associate psychosis with depression as they do for mania, a proportion of severely depressed individuals will have delusions or hallucinations during depression. The psychotic features that appear in depression often are described as "mood-congruent," meaning the content of the delusion or hallucination is in keeping with the direction of the mood—in this case, down. So if your partner is diagnosed as having severe depression with psychotic features, she might believe she is evil or possessed by the devil, or that she's experiencing some kind of physical deterioration such as her insides are rotting away and/or that she has a foul smell, that she has lost all of her money and is impoverished, or that she is being punished by God. Hallucinations tend to be less common than delusions but involve similar themes.

Research suggests that people either tend to have or not have psychotic depressions. So if your loved one has had delusions or hallucinations during past episodes of depression, he is likely to have them in subsequent full-blown, severe episodes too.

The only real treatment for psychotic features of depression is pharmacological (see Chapter 4). Therefore, it's critical that you contact the doctor immediately if you see any signs of psychosis in your partner.

How do you deal with your mate's psychosis while waiting for the medication to take effect? First, it's important to recognize that *you will not be able to convince your mate that her false perception is untrue.* By their very nature delusions are untrue but unshakable beliefs—you can't "talk" someone out of one. You may, however, be able to decrease your mate's emotional response to the delusion by providing reassurance, saying something like "I love you no matter what," "I'm here for you," or "We'll find a way to deal with this."

What about My Feelings?

It is very difficult—on a number of levels—to watch your loved one go through the torment of a depression, and you may find yourself experiencing many emotions that are atypical for you. How do you cope with these uncomfortable feelings of your own?

Confused

"I just don't get it. Everything in her life is so great."

Many people who've never experienced a depression have a hard time understanding how anyone can be so low without having experienced

Sample Contract for Suicide Prevention

If having thoughts of self-harm, my partner will:

- Share suicidal thoughts or plans with me and the doctor(s).
- Turn over any weapons.
- Give me his pills.
- Abstain from drinking or using recreational drugs.
- Seek counsel with his pastor, priest, rabbi, etc.
- Go to the hospital (if hospitalization is necessary).

If my partner is having thoughts of self-harm, I will:

- Stay with him.
- Call the doctor(s) to arrange emergency appointments.
- Remove alcohol and weapons from the home.
- Take possession of all pills.
- Drive him to the hospital (if hospitalization is necessary).

Our signatures below indicate that we agree to the above:

_____

Signature of Partner #1

_____

Signature of Partner #2

From *When Someone You Love Is Bipolar* by Cynthia G. Last. Copyright 2009 by Cynthia G. Last.

some truly traumatic event. I hope that, having read the preceding chapters in this book, you now have a better understanding of the largely biological/genetic basis of this illness and, therefore, how bipolar cycling occurs.

However, if you still find it difficult to fathom what's going on with your mate, you may benefit from attending a support group for partners of bipolar people, where you can talk to others who are in a similar situation. It also may be helpful to read one of the many excellent firsthand accounts of bipolar depression written by individuals who have suffered through it (see in particular Duke, Jamison, and Sutherland in the Resources at the back of this book).

Worried

"What if he tries to hurt himself?"

I wish I could just say you have nothing to worry about. But when you see your loved one sink to the depths that depression can bring, and you know from Chapter 2 that the suicide rate is greatly increased with bipolar disorder, being frightened is perfectly understandable. But you don't have to live in a state of terror (and, in fact, doing so would only be hard on you and your partner). You can remind yourself that there *is* a risk but that, armed as you are with both knowledge and resources, you are doing everything humanly possible to minimize the danger:

- The threat of suicide is greatest for people who are untreated, self-medicating with alcohol, and have a past history of suicide attempts. Your partner's adhering to treatment and staying away from alcohol are significant protective factors even if they can't serve as a guarantee.
- Knowing what constitutes suicide "red flags"—suicidal thinking and suspicious behavior—as described in this chapter, relieves you of agonizing over whether you might be overreacting or underreacting. Having a suicide prevention contract and an emergency plan in place means you're prepared to act the minute you do see any of those signs.
- You have professionals available to help: any suspicions you have justify an immediate call to your mate's physician. If you can't reach the doctor and you believe your partner is in imminent danger, take your partner to the emergency room. If you're left with no other recourse, call the police.

If these reminders don't reassure you that you're as prepared to protect your partner as anyone could be, you might benefit from seeking professional help for your anxiety.

Angry

"If she had taken better care of herself, she wouldn't be this way now."

Having bipolar disorder is not your partner's fault; it's largely a genetic illness. But if you're angry because you think your partner could have

done more to prevent this particular episode of depression from happening, try to remember that whether or not your partner has a recurrence is only partly in her control. Episodes of illness can recur even
with strict adherence to medication and good management of all the
lifestyle factors discussed in Chapter 7. So first, I encourage you to call
on your capacity for compassion.

On the other hand, if your partner has departed from his treatment regimen, you have a right to be upset. His actions have had a big
impact not only on your mate, but also on you and your life together.
Maybe this terrible time, though, can be in some way a learning experience for the two of you.

If your mate reduced or discontinued her medication because of
certain side effects, perhaps you and your partner need to talk to the
doctor about alternative medications that don't have the same ones.
Or if your partner's recurrence is related to poor stress management,
maybe this is a wake-up call that it's time (although not when your
partner is in the thick of the depression) for your mate—or for the two
of you together—to develop new skills for coping with stress, such as
relaxation techniques, yoga, and/or meditation (see the Resources at
the end of this book), or to make some other lifestyle changes.

What's important is to look ahead to the future, to potentially
better days informed by your knowledge of this episode and what may
have brought it on.

Sad

"I can't bear seeing him this way."

Watching someone you love suffering can be an agonizing experience.
It's hard to see your partner in pain day after day, week after week,
even possibly for months. Particularly if you are a sensitive and empathetic person, you may feel that, to some extent, you are experiencing
what your partner is going through too.

Writing about the experience, by keeping a journal, can help people clarify their feelings and put some distance between themselves
and their emotions. Talking to others who are going through the same
thing (again, a support group for you) and/or to a mental health professional can be beneficial too. Keep in mind that severe and pervasive sadness may indicate that you yourself have become depressed. In
that case, you may need a medical intervention. Consider scheduling a

medication evaluation with a physician (possibly your mate's psychiatrist, if you are comfortable with him or her and your partner doesn't have any issues with your seeing the same doctor). And also don't forget to use the strategies for depression—for yourself—in this chapter.

Lonely

"I feel like I'm living by myself."

It is very characteristic of depression for people to withdraw from others—including even their primary relationships, and to become entirely focused on themselves and their pain. As the spouse of one patient of mine put it, "Although my partner is physically present, mentally and emotionally he is not. I still have a partner, but no real partnership. I feel alone."

Although you may feel very much alone as the partner of a depressed man or woman, know that you are not alone. Thousands of spouses are going through the same experience right now. And that's why a support group can be so helpful. It's a place where you can bond with others who are experiencing the same feelings. It's also important to stay connected to your own friends and family. Even though they certainly aren't a replacement for your relationship with your partner, and they may not really understand what you are going through, their love and concern will help you to not feel so alone.

Helpless

"I don't know how to help her."

I hope the tools and strategies offered in this chapter have lessened any feelings of helplessness you've had. But if you think you need to do more because your partner doesn't seem to be improving, please remember that even with all the help you can give and the right medication, it may take weeks or even months for your loved one to return to her old self.

I was one of the fortunate ones to have a relatively quick and complete response to antidepressant medication so that I didn't suffer for too long. Other individuals don't have as fast or dramatic a reaction and actually may get somewhat worse before medication, therapy, and the "antidepressant" techniques included in this chapter come together and gradually provide relief. That's why it's important to be aware of small changes in your mate's mood and behavior while your partner is being treated for depression. Mood monitoring, discussed in Chapter 7, is a valuable tool to help you keep this perspective.

Sexually Frustrated

"It's been months since we made love."

The plain truth is that depression and lack of sexual desire go hand in hand. Consequently, it's highly unlikely that your mate is going to want to be physically intimate with you during the course of a severe depression. This is no reflection on you (although it may feel like it), but rather has to do with other factors inherent in the experience and treatment of bipolar depression:

- Your mate feels physically unattractive (old, ugly, fat) and sexually undesirable.
- Your mate feels vulnerable or fragile and can't handle intimacy right now.
- Your mate no longer pays attention to her grooming and isn't comfortable relating on a sexual basis.
- Your mate is withdrawn and wants to be left alone.
- Medication side effects have decreased your mate's sexual desire or interfered with his/her ability to achieve erection/orgasm.
- Your mate is feeling exhausted and doesn't have the energy for the exertion that sex requires.
- Your mate can't experience pleasure from anything right now, including sex.

If your sexual relationship was good before the depression, there's no reason it shouldn't continue in the same vein after your mate is well. In this case, the sexual problem you and your mate are experiencing is a symptom of bipolar illness (or its treatment), not a symptom of your relationship. But if the two of you have never had a satisfying sexual relationship, your situation will require more attention. When your mate is feeling better (*not* while depressed), you may want to broach the topic of your sexual relationship by asking him how satisfied he is with your sex life. Chances are if you aren't satisfied, he isn't either. Then, if the two of you are committed to being together and working on intimacy, you could propose that you get outside help from a health care provider who specializes in this area.

For the most part, the spouses I've met have been pretty understanding about the trouble their partners had with intimacy when depressed. They've been successful, too, at slowly resuming their romantic lives as their loved ones improved, beginning, in many cases, with small demonstrations of affection and then slowly proceeding to increasingly intimate contact.

Whether it's mania or depression, being alert to early warning signs and taking quick action to intervene will spare you and your partner the worst effects of full-blown bipolar episodes in many cases. But, unfortunately, not in all cases. If your partner has succumbed to a full episode of mania or depression, in the aftermath there will be fallout to deal with. The final chapter in this book offers suggestions for managing the practical and emotional consequences of an episode, for handling ongoing issues raised by having a relationship with someone who has this illness, and for maintaining your own health and happiness in the midst of it all.

10

Taking Care of Yourself and Your Relationship

Seeing your partner begin to stabilize after an episode of mania or depression is an enormous relief, like watching the sun emerge after a dark and destructive storm. Unfortunately, you may hardly have time to catch your breath before you have to contend with the fallout of the illness.

The aftermath of a mood episode can be as difficult to cope with as the episode itself. Cleaning up the damage can absorb all your energy, and even though you know that the situation you now face is not really your partner's fault, that it is a manifestation of the illness, you may find you're having negative feelings toward your mate.

In the end, if your relationship is to survive, you will need some way to deal with the feelings you are experiencing so that you can put the past in the past. And not only for your relationship's sake, but for your sake too, that is, for you as an individual. It's not healthy for you to be consumed with intense anxiety, anger, sadness, or other negative feelings. It's important to do what you can to preserve your relationship, but it's equally, if not more, important that you not become so consumed with your partner's illness that you end up losing yourself.

There also will be other challenges that your relationship will face because of your partner's having bipolar disorder, not just following mood episodes, but on an ongoing or intermittent basis throughout your lifetime together. Some of these will involve making very difficult decisions that will affect your future—like whether to have children. Others will involve dealing with sensitive issues that affect you both—such as trying to remedy an unfulfilling sex life. And still others will entail examining roles you may have taken on that are not beneficial to you, your partner, or your relationship. I'll help you with these, too.

If you work together, I believe you and your spouse will be able to meet the challenges that confront you. However, in the event that your situation does not improve, you may have a very difficult choice ahead of you. I'll be talking about making that decision—the decision to leave one's relationship—later on in this chapter. For now, let's start by seeing what you can do to successfully take on the issues at hand.

Surviving the Aftermath of a Mood Episode

"I'm going to have to file for bankruptcy. My wife put us into over $100,000 in debt when she was manic, and we can't get back on our feet financially. I'm incredibly angry even though I know it really wasn't her fault."

Cleaning up the financial mess your partner made during her last manic episode can take months or years. While you're getting back on your feet you may feel a tremendous amount of resentment toward your mate and also dread the possibility of a repeat during future manic periods. In addition to following the treatment plan, instituting the measures I highlighted in Chapter 8 will help protect you from further monetary problems. But that doesn't address the feelings you're having right now.

Going to a support group (see page 275) for well partners of bipolar individuals may help. Other participants may have experienced what you're going through and not only will be able to lend a sympathetic ear but also might have useful financial advice and tips.

In addition to or instead of a support group, individual therapy can help you work through the feelings you're having. Your local community mental health center provides mental health services with fees set in relation to individual families' financial circumstances, making them affordable for virtually anybody. Another economical avenue for obtaining therapy is through a university that has a graduate-level program in psychology. Many times such programs have facilities (psychological clinics or centers) through which their doctoral students provide services, under the supervision of a licensed mental health professional, as part of their training.

"They suspended my husband's license temporarily after he was arrested for drunk driving. If he doesn't get it back, I don't know what we'll do. How will he get to work? Am I going to need to drive him every day, or should I make him take public transportation?"

It's hard to know where to draw the line—what you will and will not do for your mate—in a situation like this. On one hand, you don't want to rescue your partner from the consequences of his actions but, on the other hand, you don't want to penalize him for having a psychiatric illness.

How much of an imposition will it be for you to drive your spouse to work? Is it on the way to your work, or will it significantly lengthen the time it takes you to get there? How much of an inconvenience would it be for your mate to use public transportation? Is it complicated (requiring multiple buses, trains, subways, or some combination of these), time-consuming, or in some other way very inconvenient?

Another factor you might want to consider is whether driving under the influence has been a recurrent behavior for your mate, or whether this is the first instance of this behavior. Do you think it will be beneficial—that is, will help to prevent future instances of this kind—for your partner "to feel" the consequences of his actions? If you do, and you decide not to help your mate out, what effect will this have on your relationship? Are you prepared to deal with the anger or resentment he is likely to feel toward you?

No one, including me, can answer these questions for you; only you can do this for yourself. It might help, though, to explore some of the issues I have raised before deciding what to do.

"During her last manic episode my partner cheated on me with one of her coworkers. Now I worry about her being in the same environment with this person. What if she gets manic again? Will the temptation be too much?"

Sexual infidelity can be very hard to get past. Not only can it be difficult to live with the knowledge that your partner has been intimate with another person, but you may worry (like this person) that it will happen again in the future.

Professional help can be useful for working through the thoughts and feelings you are having about what your spouse has done. But the best defense to keep this from occurring down the road is, of course, appropriate and consistent treatment. Also following the guidelines I outlined in Chapter 8 for dealing with mania will help decrease the likelihood of high-risk behavior of this kind.

In this particular situation, it would be wise to speak to your partner about how she feels being in close proximity to the person she had the affair with. Was it just a one-night fling that was inconsequential to her? Or was it a real relationship of some type, with feelings that remain? If she still has feelings for this person, is it possible for your mate to work in another department or at another location so that she has limited or no further contact with this person? Is the situation one that would justify your partner's changing jobs?

"When my wife was depressed, I had to have our daughter stay with my parents. My wife just wasn't able to take care of her, and I had to go to work, so I couldn't physically be there for her. Now my child is showing emotional problems—separation anxiety. Have we done permanent damage to her mental health?"

If your child is showing emotional or behavioral problems, the best thing to do is to get an evaluation from a mental health professional—a psychiatrist or psychologist who specializes in treating children. The doctor will diagnose your child and determine whether—and which type of—treatment is indicated. For example, your child may need individual therapy, family therapy, or some combination of the two, and/or, depending on the nature and severity of your daughter's problem, medication.

If you haven't already discussed your spouse's illness with your child, you (and, possibly, your child's therapist too, if she is in treatment) need to do so. Communicate to your youngster, in a way that's appropriate to her age and maturity level, that your mate has an illness that sometimes keeps her from being able to give all the attention and care to your child that your child needs and deserves. Also, make sure to reassure your daughter that the illness is not one that people die from, for the fear of losing a parent will make separation anxiety worse.

"It was really scary seeing my husband psychotic. Seeing him that out of control has changed the way I look at him now, even though he's better. I just can't get those awful images out of my head. There's no way I can be intimate with him, even though I know none of this was his doing."

If during your partner's recent episode of illness you saw a side of him that was very unappealing, it can be hard to get past those recollections. Fortunately, in this case, time does help to fade memories. Also having different, more recent experiences with your mate will help to replace the older ones.

In the meantime, you might want to consider talking to your mate about how you've been feeling, particularly with respect to resuming your physical relationship. Try to be sensitive and reassuring when approaching the topic. For example, you might say something like "I'm having some trouble with getting physical with you now that you're no longer ill. I just need some more time with you being well to be comfortable with being close again." Then try small steps toward resuming your physical relationship, slowly moving to increasingly intimate contact as you become more at ease with your partner.

"It's been 6 months now, but I still can't believe that my wife actually tried to kill herself. What if she tries again, or maybe even succeeds?"

It's a tragic reality that past suicidal behavior can be predictive of future suicidal behavior, so having concern in the aftermath of a suicide attempt is, to some degree, appropriate. However, you can't live your life constantly on pins and needles, waiting for it to happen again.

The best defense, of course, to preventing self-harm is to stop mood episodes *before they start*. By following the treatment plan your partner will have a good chance of staying well. It still would be wise, though, to have a contract for preventing suicide (see Chapter 9) in place, in the event your loved one does take a turn for the worse. It's also important to be vigilant for the "red flags" (again, see Chapter 9) that suggest your partner is considering hurting herself. Finally, make sure you have your emergency plan ready to go, including knowing which hospital to take your spouse to in the event that you (or someone else who is qualified) think she is a threat to herself.

Other Challenges to Your Relationship

Deciding Whether to Have Children

If your partner became ill later on in the relationship, or if his illness has worsened over time, you may have to come to terms with accepting some hard truths about the new reality of your future together. One of the most difficult of these, I think, is the possibility of never having children.

The decision of whether or not to have children can be a heartbreaking one to make. There are many factors that need to be considered in making this choice, some of which are highlighted below:

- What is the frequency and severity of your spouse's episodes? Would he be able to meet the physical and emotional needs of a child?
- Would your partner be able to manage without medication (or on limited medications) through pregnancy (and, if applicable, nursing)?
- What is your family's genetic loading for bipolar disorder (runs on both sides of the family, present in all first-degree relatives on the ill partner' side, etc.)? How will you feel if your child develops the disorder?
- Will you be okay with shouldering more of the responsibility for raising the child in the event that your spouse's illness worsens?
- Might your partner's illness be in some way harmful—directly or indirectly—to a child?
- How do you feel about the possibility of not having children? Is having a child a prerequisite for remaining in this relationship?

As I said in Chapter 2, deciding not to have children is one of the most difficult things my husband and I have ever had to do. And I'm not always 100% sure that we made the right choice—there are times when I still get tearful about what I imagine could have been (although less so as the years have passed). Thankfully, though, we've been able to have a fulfilling relationship and productive lives. Whichever way you and your mate decide to go, I sincerely hope that the two of you can find the same level of contentment.

Lack of Physical Intimacy

In Chapter 9 I talked about why your mate may experience a low libido (see page 258). Alternatively, as a consequence of bipolar illness and/or its treatment, there are many reasons why you may have lost sexual desire for your mate:

- Your partner doesn't take care of his grooming like he used to.
- She has gained a lot of weight from the medication.
- The illness is a turn-off.
- He has trouble reaching orgasm because of the medication.
- You have trouble seeing your mate as an adult partner; she seems more like your child.
- You can't trust your partner after what he did (sexually) when manic.
- Your sexual advances always are met with rejection, so you've given up trying.

As for all couples, you are entitled to have a fulfilling sexual relationship with your partner. If you are not, then it behooves you to discuss the situation with your mate, doing so in a way that's not accusatory and unlikely to make your loved one feel solely responsible for the problem.

For instance, if you're having intimacy problems because your mate had sex outside your relationship during a manic episode, you might say, "I'm having trouble getting past what you did the last time you were manic. I'm working on it, but I don't yet feel comfortable being intimate with you." You then might take small steps toward being close again, perhaps beginning with taking a bath together or giving each other massages. If you find you're having trouble even with this level of closeness, you might consider getting some outside assistance to help you put the past in the past.

If it's medication-related issues that are affecting your attraction to your mate, the two of you may want to talk to the doctor about alternative drugs that don't have these side effects. If the cause of the problem lies elsewhere, it may be best dealt with through individual and/or couple counseling or sex therapy, or some combination of these, depending on the specifics of your situation.

Assuming the Caretaker Role

Perhaps when you married your mate didn't have bipolar disorder or, if he did, neither of you knew it. You entered this relationship as most couples do, as a partnership, but as your mate has become ill, you've ended up in a caretaker-type role.

If you find you've become the caretaker, ask yourself the following questions:

- Do you really need to be doing all that you do for your mate? Are there things that you do that she could do for herself but you don't give her a chance to do?
- Is this a role you tend to assume in relationships? If so, what about the role is fulfilling for you? Are there other ways that you can meet these needs, ones that might be better for you and for your relationship?
- What does your partner do that elicits your caregiving behavior? How can you respond to these signals other than by "taking over"?
- If your partner does require some degree of care, are other resources (individuals, organizations, facilities, etc.) available, or that could be made available, that could help out and lighten your load?
- How can you help your partner be more independent? What skills can he develop that will enable him to do more on his own? How can you support the development of these skills?
- What do you do to take care of your needs (see pages 270–272)?

If your mate is very ill at times, you'll have to take on the caretaker role during those periods. Just be sure that you don't extend this level of assistance beyond what is necessary—in other words, know when to back off. If you don't, you'll end up "crippling" your spouse by making her so dependent on you that she can't manage on her own.

As or more important, by continually adopting the caretaker role you will eventually face the inevitable physical and psychological burn-out that comes from taking on too much for too long, and then you won't be in a position to help your partner at all.

How do you know when you're about to hit that wall? By checking in with yourself on a regular basis and asking yourself the following questions, you'll know when you're becoming depleted and need to take action to help yourself:

- Are you having trouble sleeping? Difficulty falling asleep, rest-less sleep, frequently waking during the night, or waking earlier than you need to in the morning?
- Are you tired much of the time, even when you do get enough sleep?
- Have you been more irritable than usual? Do little, unimport-ant things bother you more than they should?
- Are you having physical manifestations of stress—headaches, stomachaches, or back pain?
- Are you feeling sad, down, or blue? Not looking forward to things the way you used to?
- Do you have memory lapses or mental confusion? Does your mind often seem to go blank?
- Are you feeling overwhelmed with anxiety? Tense, uptight much of the time, or having panic attacks?
- Are you using food/alcohol/caffeine/cigarettes to help you cope with stress?

If you responded with a "yes" to one or more of these questions, you already may be beginning to see signs that you're doing too much. You must step back and take time to take care of *yourself*, a topic I'll be addressing further later on.

Dealing with Recurrent Treatment Noncompliance

Does your partner repeatedly become ill because he frequently reduces or discontinues medication on his own? Have you discussed this with him but to no avail?

Treatment noncompliance, as I've explained, is a common problem among individuals who have bipolar disorder. If the noncompliance stems from medication side effects, then your mate needs to talk to her doctor about other treatment options. If the lack of adherence is related to another issue—for example, denial of the illness or the desire for manic/hypomanic episodes—then you may have no other option than to give your loved one an ultimatum (see Chapter 6).

No one can have a meaningful relationship with someone who is manic or depressed much of the time. It's not fair to you, nor is it in the best interest of your spouse. Sometimes a hard-line approach is the only thing that will work. And if it doesn't, you, unfortunately, may have an extremely difficult decision to make about the viability of your relationship, discussed later in this chapter.

Handling the Verbal Abuse

Bipolar people can be emotionally volatile even when they aren't in mood episodes (and even more so when they are), especially if they are not medicated or are medicated inadequately. It can be hard to maintain consistent loving feelings for a person who can turn on you on a dime. Of course, making sure your partner is on her optimal medication regimen should lessen this problem. The rest really is up to your spouse.

Often bipolar individuals are selective in their verbal attacks. They may be able to control this behavior in certain situations where it would be a real problem, such as with an employer. If your partner can control himself with others, then he should, theoretically, also be able to do so with you too. You will, however, need to call your mate on it when he is out of line. For example, you might say something like "I no longer will allow you to speak to me in this way." Then, if the verbal abuse continues, leave the room. By doing this you'll be firmly standing your ground.

It also may be helpful to keep in mind that when your spouse is verbally abusive it's the illness talking, not your loved one. Of course, this is easier said than done. If you can't do it and you are often deeply hurt by your partner's negative or nasty comments about you or your relationship, you have some very difficult decisions to make. We all have our limits for what we are willing to accept in a relationship, and you need to know where you draw the line. Consider giving your mate an ultimatum. Sometimes this motivates people to try harder to turn things around.

Taking Care of Your Needs

It's not unusual for psychologists (like me) to ask people whether they are taking care of their needs. I think that many men and women, though, are so busy in their day-to-day lives that they really don't spend much time reflecting on what their needs may be. That's why I begin this section by asking you to give some thought to what is most important for your happiness and well-being.

Look at the list below. After reviewing it, fill in any other needs that are important to you, ones I haven't included, at the bottom of the page. Then prioritize the list by assigning a numerical score to each item, using a "1" to indicate your most important need, a "2" designating your second most important one, and so on, until you've given a rating to each of them.

What Are My Needs?

Rank order the list of needs below by placing a "1" next to the most important need, a "2" next to the second most important need, and so on, using a "10" to designate the one that is least important to you.

To be physically fit
To feel connected to and supported by other people
To have a spiritual connection
To pursue my interests and hobbies
To be intellectually stimulated
To be productive at home, school, or work
To feel loved
To have a fulfilling sex life
To give of myself to others
To take care of my physical appearance

_____

_____

_____

_____

_____

Now that you have identified what needs are most important to you, take some time to think about whether they are being met, starting with the one you've designated as most important ("1"). For example, if your number one need is to give of yourself to others, do you feel this need is being fully (or at least fully enough) met? Perhaps you give of yourself to your partner, friends, and family, but you would feel a deeper sense of satisfaction if you contributed more to your community or an organization that's important to you? Or, using another example, if a need that's high on your list is to be intellectually stimulated, what activities are you involved in that challenge your intellect? If a spiritual connection is a priority, how are you meeting this need? Are you satisfied with your place of worship (if you participate in organized religion), or should you be exploring others that might be a better fit for you? If you feel you are significantly lacking in the area of spirituality but would like to rectify this, what steps can you take to bring you closer to this goal?

If your answer to the exercise above is to say "I don't have time to focus on my needs, the demands on me from my partner and everything else take up all my time," then you are one of the people for whom this activity is largely designed. Answer this question: "Am I completely happy and fulfilled in my life?" If your answer is "yes," then go ahead and skip the exercise, but if your answer is "no," I suggest you reconsider and spend some time examining the issues that have been raised here.

An important need of mine is:

_____

_____

How I currently am meeting this need:

_____

_____

_____

Other things I could do to further meet this need:

_____

_____

_____

_____

_____

_____

A strong need of mine is to be productive. Although my practice is a great source of satisfaction to me—giving of myself, improving the health of others, enhancing my self-esteem by demonstrating my expertise, providing intellectual stimulation—it doesn't, per se, produce a "product." Which is, I think, one reason I find it so rewarding to write books, which provide very tangible end products of one's efforts.

You Need Support Too

Time and again I've found in my work with the well spouses of bipolar patients that they need as much support as (if not more than) their mates. What constitutes emotional support varies from person to person, however. Some people find it most helpful just to have someone to *listen* to what they have to say. Although I am not a psychoanalytically oriented therapist, I know from experience that for many people the expression of intense emotions seems to lessen them ("catharsis"), making them more manageable.

Others welcome help with *solving problems* that arise. Members of your inner circle—the group of people you can depend on for support—may have a fresh perspective on a situation you've been wrestling with or may have better problem-solving skills than you currently do (see Chapter 7 for more on problem solving).

Some individuals benefit most from the *resources* others make available to them. Having a friend bring over a casserole (so you don't

---

Your Circle of Support

Whom can you count on to be a *sympathetic listener*?

1. _____

2. _____

3. _____

Whom can you count on to help you *solve problems* that arise?

1. _____

2. _____

3. _____

Whom can you count on to help by *providing resources* to you?

1. _____

2. _____

3. _____

From *When Someone You Love Is Bipolar* by Cynthia G. Last. Copyright 2009 by Cynthia G. Last.

---

have to cook dinner) on a day when you've encountered many stresses can feel like a lifesaver. Or if your mate is very ill and should not be left alone, some members of your inner circle may be willing to fill in for you when you need a break.

To some extent the degree to which you will need emotional support depends on the course of your loved one's illness. If your mate has symptoms much of the time, has very severe mood episodes, or has impaired day-to-day functioning, you probably will need more support than, say, someone married to a person who has a much milder form of bipolar disorder.

Where to Turn?

Whom can you turn to and count on for support? How can you tell who will be understanding, reassuring, and supportive and who will be negative and unhelpful, perhaps even hurtful, when you share what's going on with your partner?

You might assume that people who love and care for you will be able to give you what you need in the way of comfort and support. I have to tell you, though, that this is not always the case. Some people are just not psychologically minded, others are uncomfortable dealing with other people's emotional pain, and others just—for whatever reason—don't seem to have the time to devote to giving support (see the sidebar below).

In assessing someone's ability to be supportive, it's best to start out testing the water by sharing just a little bit of what you've been experiencing. Begin with friends or family members you suspect will be good sources of support—for example, people whom you know (from past behavior) to be very caring or those who have had mental health problems of their own or in their own families. Keep in mind, though, that the best people to turn to may not necessarily be those who are closest to you or your mate. Don't fall into the "but it's his/her mother/father/brother/sister/best friend" trap. The fact that someone

People You Should *Not* Turn To

"The Disbelievers"

"There's no such thing as manic–depression."
"I don't believe in psychiatrists and psychologists."
"People with psychiatric disorders are just weak."

"The Fortune-Tellers"

"He's never going to get better."
"Suicide is a sin; she's going to hell."
"That medication isn't going to work."

"The Avoiders"

"Let's talk about something else."
"Why don't you just leave him?"
"I'll come visit you when she's feeling better."

loves your spouse (or you) doesn't necessarily mean that she can be supportive.

If after confiding in someone you find that the response (or lack of response) leaves you feeling worse than before, take that as a sign that this probably isn't an individual who can play a supportive role for you. Don't continue to try to get someone to respond to your needs who, the evidence suggests, isn't capable of doing so; you'll only be disappointed repeatedly.

As I've discussed in other chapters, there are ways to get the support you need other than relying on friends and relatives. There are support groups for the loved ones of bipolar patients that can give you an outlet for sharing your experiences (and learning from others too!). Be aware, though, as you probably know now from having read this book, that there is a very wide spectrum of severity when it comes to bipolar illness. If you find you can't relate to the members of a particular support group because their circumstances are so different from yours, see if you can find another that better meets your needs. Also, if you can't find a bipolar support group, consider attending one for caregivers. Even though the illnesses participants have to deal with are different, the challenges that come can be the same.

You also can connect with other partners of bipolar people through the Internet—many of the bipolar disorder websites (see Resources) have forums that enable people (bipolar individuals, partners) to communicate with each other. This may be an especially good choice if you live far away from where the nearest group meets.

Your place of worship—either the clergy or parishioners or both—may be another resource. But don't assume, because you share the same faith and frequent the same church or synagogue, that these individuals will be sympathetic to your situation. Test the water with them just as I recommend you do with friends and family.

Consider visiting a mental health professional. Not only are these individuals trained to deal with problems like those you're experiencing, but you won't need to be concerned about possibly "burdening" or "overwhelming" them with your situation (as you might with a friend or family member). While on this note, I also want to mention the importance of not overloading any one individual (other than a mental health professional) with your need for support. If at all possible, it's best to seek support from several different people so that any one friend or relative doesn't become as overtaxed as you sometimes feel.

Supporting Yourself

I realize that some of you reading this will not be comfortable with the idea of turning to others and sharing what you are going through. Although I really do believe there are benefits to opening up to another individual, some people just find it "unnatural" or "unseemly" to do this. If you are one of these people, you may prefer to provide your own "support" by using various techniques to destress.

The following list is just a sampling of the kinds of activities you can try to gain some peace and to replenish your personal resources:

Physical activity (exercise, sports)
Socializing with friends
Relaxation exercises
Listening to music
Yoga
Meditation
Pursuing a favorite hobby
Aromatherapy
A hot bath or shower
Reading a good book
Getting a massage

This list may seem pretty simplistic if you feel overwhelmed by loving and living with someone who has bipolar disorder. I'm not suggesting that taking a hot bath is a panacea for the stress that may seem like a permanent resident in your life. I'm not saying that, when you're filled with sadness watching your partner struggle or overflowing with frustration over the difficulties imposed on your life together, a cup of coffee with a friend is going to change your entire outlook. What I am saying is that each of these pursuits, when incorporated into your life *on a regular basis*, can to some degree alleviate whatever level of chronic stress you experience. I'm saying that I hope you'll start tuning in to your own well-being every day and take measures to be good to yourself in whatever small way you can afford.

Maybe you don't feel like you can take an hour and a half to go to the gym every day, but could you spend 20 minutes on a brisk walk through the park? Physical activity of almost any kind, to almost any degree—exercise, sports, etc.—can reduce anxiety and improve your mood. Regular exercise will make you sleep better and feel stronger. Maybe model building or scrapbooking seems kind of trivial in the face of the challenges you're dealing with. But pursuing activities that you love—your hobbies or interests—can be very rejuvenating, and deciding to allot a certain amount of time per week to these endeavors is like putting money in the form of energy and positive attitude in the bank. You may never have thought of yourself as the type to meditate or do yoga. But if you try it, you might discover that relaxation exercises, yoga, and meditation can decrease anxiety and increase your ability to handle stress. There are items on the list above that you can make a regular part of your life, and there are others that you can resolve to turn to as the need arises.

Space does not allow me to go into detail about any of these techniques and other outlets, but there are many sources of instruction and information that you can turn to; I've listed some of them in the Resources section at the back of this book.

When Enough Is Enough

"Sometimes I feel I can't go on this way anymore. I know that I made a commitment to this person, but I don't think it's fair for me to have to spend the rest of my life this way. But then I think, 'She doesn't want to be like this,' and I feel guilty for even considering leaving. After all, what would she do without me? Who would take care of her?"

Being married to a person with bipolar disorder, it's fairly safe to assume you've had times where you've seriously questioned whether you might be better off without the relationship. Relationships, even for couples who don't have to contend with mental health problems, are difficult; bipolar illness increases that level of difficulty, particularly when it's untreated or treated inadequately.

Are you basically happy? If not, does a large part of your discontent stem from problems in your relationship? Where are the problems in the relationship? Is change likely? How long are you willing to wait for change (6 months, 1 year, 5 years, a lifetime)? Sometimes you need to ask yourself hard questions like these. Although it can be difficult to face the truth, nothing will change unless you first acknowledge what is wrong.

What currently is lacking from our relationship (for example, companionship, fulfilling sex life, love, affection, intellectual stimulation, joy and laughter, a sense of stability)?

_____

_____

_____

_____

Which of the above has to change for me to remain in this relationship?

_____

_____

_____

_____

How can I help to effect these changes? (*List specific things you can do.*)

_____

_____

_____

_____

What can my partner do to help effect these changes? (*List specific things your partner can do.*)

_____

_____

_____

_____

Patsy and Fernando haven't had sex in several years. At first, Patsy blamed it on her depression. But the depression ended nearly 2 years ago, and she still comes up with excuses to avoid being intimate with her husband. Fernando has spoken to Patsy about the possibility of both of them together seeing a therapist to work on this problem, but Patsy outright refuses. She says, "Sex just isn't important to me anymore."

It's possible that Patsy's decreased sexual interest is a side effect of one of her medications. If she and her husband can trace the onset of the problem to the time period when she began a particular medication, they might be able to identify which of the drugs is causing the problem. Then Patsy could talk to her doctor about the possibility of trying another medication—one that doesn't have sexual side effects—in its place.

But what if Patsy's lack of desire is not a medication side effect but has deeper roots, ones she's unwilling to look at or address? Does Fernando accept the absence of a sex life with his partner? Does he go outside the relationship to meet his needs? Or does he call it quits with his wife?

Like Fernando, Matt has difficult questions he must ask himself. Simone developed rapid-cycling bipolar disorder last year, about 6 months after they got engaged. The problem is that she refuses to be treated for her illness, or even to work on her own to try to help stabilize her mood swings. Does Matt go through with the wedding? What are the chances that Simone will "wake up" and do what she needs to do for her mental health? Is this too much of a gamble?

Matt's friends and relatives have a lot of different opinions about what he should do. Some of them feel he should definitely "get out" while he can. Others downplay the situation, saying that having bipolar disorder really is "no big deal" and shouldn't play a role in making his decision. But, in the end, Matt really has to listen to his own head and heart. He's got to be honest with himself about his own capabilities. He needs to evaluate whether he will be able, when necessary, to play a caregiver role, and whether he is the type of person who can be supportive without giving up himself altogether. When he asks himself these questions, and considers his feelings for his partner, he wants to go through with the wedding. But he wants Simone to do her part too, so he gives her an ultimatum—the marriage will be postponed until she gets treatment for her illness (see Chapter 6 for how to give an ultimatum).

Maybe, like the person I quoted at the beginning of this section, you want to end your relationship but you feel you don't really have a choice, that you are "trapped" because your mate is ill and dependent on you and there is no one else to take over this responsibility. But, in reality, there always are choices. If your partner can't live on his or her own, there may be relatives who can step in. If not, there are alternative living situations ("transitional" living facilities) for people with chronic mental illnesses who can't live entirely on their own.

Or, maybe, although it would be feasible for you to leave the relationship, you feel you couldn't do it because you would be filled with guilt. You think, "What kind of person leaves a sick spouse?" When you married, you vowed "for better or worse, in sickness and in health." You want to live up to those vows, but what price are you willing to pay? If your partner hasn't changed, and you anticipate she is unlikely to do so in the future, are you willing to devote the rest of your life to her? What about you and what you want and need?

I wish I could help you more, but, of course, I don't know your specific situation. Even if I did, I wouldn't be able to make the decision for you. Only you can do this through what I know will be much soul searching. You also may want to talk to a person you've turned to and trusted in the past when really difficult choices have come up—a friend, a family member, a mental health professional. Not to ask the other person what to do, but just to be a sounding board. Sometimes proposing what you're thinking out loud instantly makes you realize it's right or wrong.

If you do find you are at the end of the road in your relationship—that you've tried everything you can think of to help but to no avail—please forgive yourself for deciding to end the relationship. Leave knowing that you've done your best and couldn't possibly expect yourself to do any more. That's all anyone can ask of himself.

A Final Note

A key question that's included by psychologists in assessing people's happiness in their marriages is "If you had to do it over, knowing what you know now, would you marry the same person again?" If the answer to the question is "no," it's (obviously) an indicator of dissatisfaction, while responding "yes" signifies satisfaction.

So I decided, while preparing to write this chapter, that I'd ask my husband this very telling question, prefacing it with "Now, I know how difficult it has been for you at times being with someone with bipolar disorder, so I'd understand if you answer 'no.'" But the speed of my husband's response (it was "yes," by the way), along with the assuredness with which he answered me, was startling. He didn't even have to take time to contemplate this. Despite all we'd been through over the past two decades, he was that sure he'd choose me as a life partner again.

Quite frankly, if I were in his position, I don't know that I would have answered in the same way. I don't know that I could meet the challenges that go along with having a bipolar spouse. But, then, I'm not my husband. I work to make things more even-keeled in my life, while my husband, on the other hand, who by nature is very steady, likes things stirred up a little. In that way, we complement each other. He enjoys the spontaneous, witty, creative, passionate, bubbly aspects of my personality, while I cherish his steadfastness and, yes, predictability.

From the many spouses of bipolar people I have met in my practice, I know that a lot of you reading this are like my husband. Given the chance, you'd pick the same partner again. And that's because as much as bipolar disorder presents very real obstacles, your mate has special qualities, the qualities that made you fall in love with him or her.

When times get tough, remember those qualities. And when times are not as tough, enjoy each other and your lives together. You've both worked hard to keep the bipolar beast at bay. Rejoice in your successes. The two of you deserve it.

Resources

Selected Books on Bipolar Disorder

Duke, P., and Turan, K. (1987). *Call me Anna*. New York: Bantam Books.

Fieve, R. R. (1997). *Moodswing*. New York: Bantam Books.

Goodwin, F. K., and Jamison, K. R. (2007). *Manic–depressive illness*. New York: Oxford University Press.

Holloway, A. A. (2006). *The bipolar bear family: When a parent has bipolar disorder*. New York: AuthorHouse.

Jamison, K. R. (1995). *An unquiet mind*. New York: Knopf.

Miklowitz, D. J. (2002). *The bipolar disorder survival guide*. New York: Guilford Press.

Mondimore, F. M. (1999). *Bipolar disorder: A guide for patients and families*. Baltimore: Johns Hopkins University Press.

Sutherland, S. (1998). *Breakdown*. New York: Oxford University Press.

Torrey, E. F., and Knable, M. B. (2002). *Surviving manic–depression*. New York: Basic Books.

Books That Offer Help with Related Problems

RELAXATION EXERCISES

Barlow, D. H., and Craske, M. G. (2006). *Mastery of your anxiety and panic: Workbook*. New York: Oxford University Press.

Bourne, E. J. (2005). *The anxiety and phobia workbook*. Oakland, CA: New Harbinger.

Davis, M., Eshelman, E. R., and McKay, M. (2008). *The relaxation and stress reduction workbook*. Oakland, CA: New Harbinger.

CHANGING UNHELPFUL THOUGHTS AND BELIEFS

Beck, A. T. (1988). *Love is never enough: How couples can overcome misunderstandings, resolve conflicts, and solve relationship problems through cognitive therapy*. New York: HarperCollins.

Burns, D. D. (1999). *Feeling good: The new mood therapy*. New York: Avon Books.

Craske, M. G., and Barlow, D. H. (2006). *Mastery of your anxiety and worry: Workbook*. New York: Oxford University Press.

McKay, M., and Fanning, P. (2000). *Self-esteem: A proven program of cognitive techniques for assessing, improving, and maintaining your self-esteem*. Oakland, CA: New Harbinger.

MEDITATION

Davich, V. (2004). *8 minute meditation: Change your mind, change your life*. New York: Penguin Books.

Gunaratana, B. H. (2002). *Mindfulness in plain English*. Somerville, MA: Wisdom.

Kabat-Zinn, J. (1994). *Wherever you go there you are: Mindfulness meditation in everyday life*. New York: Hyperion.

Williams, M., Teasdale, J., Segal, Z., and Kabat-Zinn, J. (2007). *The mindful way through depression: Freeing yourself from chronic unhappiness*. New York: Guilford Press.

Internet Resources

(Sites that are <u>underlined</u> are especially geared toward spouses and partners.)

About.Com: Bipolar Disorder
www.bipolar.about.com

This site contains a lot of information about the illness and also has three chat "bulletin boards" for people to communicate on regarding specific topics pertinent to bipolar disorder.

Bipolar Disorder Web
www.bipolardisorderweb.com

In addition to the usual information on bipolar disorder, this site
contains numerous postings by significant others of bipolar individuals on
relationship issues.

Bipolar Meetup Groups
www.bipolar.meetup.com

This site enables bipolar individuals to locate "meet-up" groups near them—
currently, there are groups in the United States, Canada, Great Britain, and
Ireland—for discussion, information, and support.

Bipolar News Org
www.bipolarnews.org

This site includes the latest news on bipolar disorder research (and on major
depression too), including abstracts from actual journal articles. This is
an incredibly valuable resource for people who want to stay up-to-date on
what's happening in the field.

Bipolar Significant Other Mailing List
www.bpso.org

In addition to the helpful material presented on this site, there is a "mailing
list" for members (membership is open to significant others of bipolar
individuals who don't have the illness themselves) so they can e-mail and
exchange information, support, and discuss the impact the illness has on
their relationships.

Bipolar Support Org
www.bipolarsupport.org

The purpose of this site is to provide information and to offer support, not
only to those with bipolar illness, but to the family, loved ones, and friends
of those afflicted. The site includes many supportive forums and chat
rooms; overall, it creates a real community-like atmosphere.

Bipolar World
www.bipolarworld.net

As outlined in its mission statement, the primary purpose of this site is to
provide a safe, interactive self-help environment for individuals with bipolar

disorder to meet, share, and support each other. There also is a fair amount of material on this site geared to spouses and partners.

Bipolar 4 All
www.bipolar4all.co.uk

This U.K. site describes itself as a safe haven for anyone—including family and friends—touched by bipolar disorder. It offers information and support, including useful links for caregivers.

Fyreniyce
www.members.iinet.net.au/~fractal1

When you first enter Australia's premier bipolar website, Fyreniyce, you are immediately struck by its visual "edginess." Once you get past this, the site contains a lot of helpful information presented in a user-friendly manner, an e-mail support group, and a real-time support group.

Harbor of Refuge Organization, Inc.
www.harbor-of-refuge.org

The site offers peer-to-peer support for people with bipolar disorder and for those—family members and friends—who care about them (right now, there are several discussions scheduled that address family and relationship issues). The site has a very friendly community feel to it.

Living Bipolar
www.livingbipolar.co.nz

The purpose of this New Zealand site is to provide up-to-date information and support to the 20,000 people who live in the country with bipolar disorder, as well as raise awareness of the disorder in the wider community.

McMan's Depression and Bipolar Web
www.mcmanweb.com

This is a very sophisticated, informative website developed by the man who is behind the well-known bipolar newsletter (you can sign up to receive the newsletter here).

Pendulum Resources
www.pendulum.org

Since 1994, *pendulum.org* has been the Web's premium resource for bipolar information. Take one look and you'll see why. It's extraordinarily comprehensive, including information not contained on most other websites (recent books, upcoming conferences, latest news).

Organizations

UNITED STATES

Child and Adolescent Bipolar Foundation
www.bpkids.org

The foundation is a parent-led, not-for-profit, Web-based organization of families raising children and teens with, or at risk for, bipolar disorder. To take advantage of its services, you have to become a member—either "family" or "professional"—by making a small donation to the foundation. Some helpful features include online support groups for parents and a "find-a-doctor" listing of the organization's professional members by state/province.

Depression and Bipolar Support Alliance
www.dbsalliance.org

The mission of the alliance is to improve the lives of people living with depression and bipolar disorder. Activities of the organization include peer-led support groups, an interactive website, educational brochures, and outreach and training programs. One of the interesting features of the website (there are many) is its inclusion of information on current clinical research trials for bipolar disorder.

International Society for Bipolar Disorders
www.isbd.org

The mission of the ISBD is to foster awareness of bipolar disorder in society at large, among mental health professionals, and to promote scientific investigation of the disorder, including international research collaboration. The official journal of the society is *Bipolar Disorders—An International Journal of Psychiatry and Neurosciences*.

National Alliance for Mental Illness
www.nami.org

NAMI is the largest grassroots organization in the United States for people with mental illness and their families. Its mission is to provide support, education, and advocacy. In addition to its website, the alliance has a helpline: 1-800-950-6264.

National Alliance for Research on Schizophrenia and Depression
www.narsad.org

NARSAD is the largest provider of funds for bipolar disorder research outside the federal government. Even though the site is for a research organization, it's very friendly and easy to navigate. If you're interested, see the summaries of recent research that's been conducted on bipolar disorder.

National Institute of Mental Health
www.nimh.nih.gov

NIMH is the largest scientific organization in the world dedicated to research focusing on mental disorders. Although there is a lot of information on bipolar disorder, it can be hard to locate, given the overwhelming nature of this site. I do, however, like the year-by-year summary of "science news"—if you also like that sort of thing, you might glance through the listing for news related to bipolar disorder.

AUSTRALIA

Australasian Society for Bipolar Disorders
www.bipolardisorders.com.au

The purpose of the society is to become the Australasian—and an internationally recognized—forum to foster ongoing collaboration, education, research, and advances in all aspects of bipolar disorder. Membership is open to mental health professionals and interested lay groups and individuals. The next conference of the group is scheduled for October 2009.

Black Dog Institute
www.blackdoginstitute.org.au

The Institute, attached to the Prince of Wales Hospital and affiliated with the University of New South Wales, is an educational, research, clinical, and community-oriented facility dedicated to improving the understanding, diagnosis, and treatment of mood disorders. It performs detailed diagnostic assessments and formulates treatment plans for bipolar patients who previously haven't responded to treatment or who have had only partial responses.

Even Keel: Bipolar Disorder Support Association
www.evenkeel.org.au

Even Keel offers a network of peer-run support groups in Western Australia to people with bipolar disorder, as well as their families and friends. There also is an online forum on its website.

SANE Australia
www.sane.org

A national charitable organization working to better the lives of people with major mental illnesses, including bipolar disorder and schizophrenia, through advocacy, education, and research support. In addition to its website, the organization has a telephone helpline that provides information and referrals.

CANADA

Mood Disorders Association of British Columbia
www.mdabc.net

The mission of the association is to provide support and education to people with mood disorders and their families and friends. MDA support groups meet in numerous locations throughout British Columbia.

Mood Disorders Association of Manitoba
www.depression.mb.ca

The association operates throughout the province of Manitoba and supports those affected by mood disorders, and their friends, families, and caregivers. Activities include peer support, public education, and advocacy.

Mood Disorders Association of Ontario
www.mooddisorders.on.ca

The association helps people with bipolar disorder and depression and their families throughout the province of Ontario with educational services, peer support groups, and telephone support.

Mood Disorders Society of Canada
www.mooddisorderscanada.ca

MDSC is a national, not-for-profit, volunteer-driven, Web-based organization that is committed to improving the quality of life for people with depression and bipolar disorder. Among the many features contained on this site, there is a comprehensive system for finding mental health services by the province and region where you live.

NEW ZEALAND

Balance NZ: Bipolar and Depression Network
www.balance.org.nz

Balance NZ is a charitable trust whose missions are support, education, advocacy, and training of New Zealanders who have bipolar disorder or major depression. In addition to support services provided for those afflicted with these illnesses, the trust offers online support groups for spouses and family members.

Bipolar Support Canterbury
www.bipolarsupportcanterbury.org.nz

A not-for-profit charity; this organization's members consist of those afflicted with bipolar disorder, their families, and supportive health professionals. The focus of the group is on meeting the needs of people in the city of Christchurch, including providing information about the disorder, running peer support groups, providing one-on-one support, and conducting information and education sessions.

UNITED KINGDOM

Bipolar Carers Trust UK—Wales
www.bipolarcarerstrustuk.co.uk

A registered charity based in Wales that runs free 2-day courses for small groups of carers of bipolar individuals in both Wales and England. The course—"Together"—is designed to increase carers' ability to cope and to support their loved ones more effectively.

Bipolar Fellowship Scotland
www.bipolarscotland.org.uk

Bipolar Fellowship Scotland is a membership organization whose aims are to provide information, support, and advice for people affected by bipolar disorder and for all those who care, to promote self-help throughout Scotland, and to educate about the illness and the organization.

Equilibrium: The Bipolar Foundation
www.bipolar-foundation.org

An independent, international, nongovernmental organization (charitable, nonprofit) dedicated to improving treatment and understanding the causes and effects of bipolar disorder. Its launch originally was hosted by Oxford

University in the United Kingdom. From what I can gather from the site, this is mostly an advocacy group aimed at decreasing prejudice and stigma associated with the illness around the globe.

MDF: The Bipolar Disorder Organization
www.mdf.org.uk

Established in 1983, this national, user-led charitable organization is for people whose lives are affected by bipolar disorder, enabling members to take advantage of its services, including self-help groups, employment advice, information and publications, a self-management program, travel insurance, and a 24-hour legal advice line. The organization also works to combat the stigma and prejudice experienced by those with the illness.

Mood Swings Network
www.moodswings.org.uk

A mental health charity, this organization offers free and confidential information, advice, and support to people with bipolar disorder and depression, carers, and health and social care professionals, from all around the United Kingdom. There currently are specific support services for carers, including a "Carers Support Group" and "Carers Pamper Day."

Index

Abilify, 101. *See also* Atypical
    antipsychotics; Medication
Abuse, verbal, 228, 269–270
"Accelerated mode," 14, 15
Acceptance of the diagnosis, 63. *See also*
    Denial of the diagnosis
Accidents, mortality rates and, 58–59.
    See also Driving
Addiction. *See* Substance abuse/use
Addison's disease, 48
Affairs, extramarital. *See* Infidelity
Age-related factors
    age at the start of illness and the
        course of the illness, 49–50
    frequency of mood episodes and,
        34–35
Agitation, 15
Alanon, 192
Alcohol use. *See also* Substance abuse/
    use
    depressive episodes and, 248–249
    driving and, 215–217
    manic or hypomanic episode and,
        217–218
    preventing mood episodes and,
        188–193
    suicide and, 57–58
Alcoholics Anonymous (AA), 191, 192
Americans with Disabilities Act, 233
An Unquiet Mind (Jamison), 65
Anger
    borderline personality disorder and,
        28
    during mania and hypomania, 11
    overview, 3
    taking care of yourself and, 227,
        255–256

Anticonvulsants, 98–101. *See also*
    Medication
Antidepressants. *See also* Medication
    list of, 109
    manic–depression "switch" and, 47
    overview, 106–109
    rapid cycling and, 47
    side effects of, 107–108
Antipsychotics, 104–106. *See also*
    Atypical antipsychotics; Medication
Anxiety
    cognitive-behavioral therapy and, 117
    sleep disturbances and, 183–185
    taking care of yourself and, 230
Anxiety disorders, 55
Appetite changes, 18
Ativan, 111. *See also* Benzodiazepines;
    Medication
Attention-deficit/hyperactivity disorder
    (ADHD), 193
Atypical antipsychotics, 101–106. *See
    also* Medication
Auditory hallucinations, 222–225. *See
    also* Hallucinations

Behavioral contract
    complete, 226
    depression and, 254
    mania and, 207, 217, 225–226
    overview, 207, 209, 225
    Sample Contract for Suicide
        Prevention form, 254
    suicide and, 252, 264–265
Beliefs
    cognitive-behavioral therapy and, 116
    expectations of yourself and, 140
Benefits of bipolar disorder, 59–60

Benzodiazepines, 110–111. *See also* Medication
Bipolar overview, 39. *See also* Course of bipolar disorder
    age and, 32, 34–35, 49–50
    benefits of bipolar disorder, 59–60
    gender and, 50–51
    statistics regarding, 2
    symptoms of, 12–21
    women and bipolar, 53
Blame
    children of people with bipolar disorder and, 4
    denial of the diagnosis and, 68, 73–76
    in depressive states, 19
    expectations of your partner's therapy and doctors and, 135–138, 137–138
    externalizing, 8, 73–76
    genetic factors in bipolar disorder and, 4
    when your partner blames you, 73–75
Books to read. *See also* Resources
    denial of the diagnosis and, 65
    list of, 283–284
Borderline personality disorder
    dialectical behavior therapy and, 118–120
    overview, 28
Boundary setting. *See also* Taking care of yourself
    expectations of yourself and, 139–140
    overview, 127–128
Breakthrough episodes, 34
Breathing exercises, 184–185
Burnout, 267–268. *See also* Taking care of yourself

Call Me Anna (Duke), 65
Cardiovascular disease, 56–57
Caretaker role, relationship with your partner and, 267–268
CBT (cognitive-behavioral therapy), 115–118
Charting of moods. *See* Mood charting; Mood monitoring
Cheating on the relationship
    dealing with after the mood episode has ended, 262–263
    during a manic or hypomanic episode, 218–219
Checklists. *See* Forms/worksheets/checklists
Children
    deciding whether you should have or not, 3–4, 52–53, 265–266

genetic factors in bipolar disorder and, 3–4, 52–53, 265–266
    after a mood episode, 263–264
    parenting during a manic or hypomanic episode, 219–220
    therapy for, 263–264
Children with bipolar disorder, age at the start of illness and, 50
Chronicity of bipolar disorder, 67–68
Cigarette smoking, cardiovascular disease and, 56
Clozaril, 101–102. *See also* Atypical antipsychotics; Medication
Codependence, 139. *See also* Taking care of yourself
Cognitive-behavioral therapy (CBT), 115–118
Communication skills
    cognitive-behavioral therapy and, 117
    conflict resolution and, 193–198
    with someone who is depressed, 247
    with someone who is hypomanic, 208
    with someone who is manic, 221
Conflict resolution, 193–198
Confusion, taking care of yourself and, 253–254
Contract, behavioral. *See* Behavioral contract
Core mindfulness skills, 119. *See also* Mindfulness
Course of bipolar disorder
    age and, 32, 34–35, 49–50
    age at the start of illness and, 49–50
    benefits of bipolar disorder, 59–60
    duration of mood episodes, 36–39
    frequency of mood episodes and, 33–36
    gender and, 50–54
    in between mood episodes, 39–42
    mortality rates and, 56–59
    other disorders that are similar to bipolar and, 54–56
    overview, 31–32
    triggers of mood episodes, 42–49
Coworkers, telling about the condition and, 233
Creativity, as a benefit of bipolar disorder, 59–60
Cushing's disease, 48
Cycling. *See also* Frequency of mood episodes
    age and, 34–35, 50
    medication and, 33–34

rapid, 34–35, 47, 51
treatment and, 33–34
Cyclothymic disorder, 22–23
Cytomel, 114

DBT (dialectical behavior therapy),
    118–120
Death, thinking about. *See* Suicidal
    thoughts or behaviors
Decision making
    avoid major decisions during
        depressive episodes and, 243
    avoid major decisions during manic or
        hypomanic episode and, 211
    cognitive-behavioral therapy and, 117
    in depressive states, 19
    warning signs of a depressive episode
        and, 243
    warning signs of a manic or
        hypomanic episode and, 211
Deep muscle relaxation, 184–185
Delusions. *See also* Psychotic features
    atypical antipsychotics and, 101
    depressive episodes and, 252–253
    how to talk to your delusional partner,
        214, 222
    manic episodes and, 221–222
    in manic versus hypomanic episodes,
        12
    overview, 221–222
    safety and, 220–225
    schizoaffective disorder and, 27
    schizophrenia and, 26–27
Denial of the diagnosis
    forgetting to take medication and,
        155
    how denial looks, 69–84
    normalization as, 70–73
    overview, 61–64
    persistence of, 84–85
    reasons for, 64–69
    relationship with your partner and,
        268–269
    self-help books and, 169
Depakote, 98–100. *See also*
    Anticonvulsants; Medication; Mood
    stabilizers
Dependence, 140–142
Depression
    cognitive-behavioral therapy and,
        115–118
    cyclothymic disorder and, 22–23
    denial of the diagnosis and, 80–83
    discussing treatment during, 71

double depression, 40
early intervention plan and, 242–248
early warning signs of, 237–241
helping your partner deal with,
    235–259
medical treatment for, 111–114
misdiagnosis of, 21, 24–26
overview, 11–12, 236–237
postpartum period and, 51–52
psychotic features and, 252–253
seasonal affective disorder and, 23
seasonal patterns of, 44–45
substance use and, 49
suicide and, 57–58
symptoms of, 17–20
taking care of yourself and, 253–259
women and bipolar and, 53
Diagnosis of bipolar. *See also* Denial of
    the diagnosis
    cyclothymic disorder, 22–23
    major depressive disorder and, 24–26
    manic and hypomanic episodes and,
        12
    misdiagnosis and, 21, 24–26
    mixed episodes and, 20–21, 24–26
    obtaining and accepting, 9
    other disorders that are similar to
        bipolar and, 26–30
    substance abuse and, 29–30
    type I and type II bipolar disorder,
        21–22
    your role in, 24–25
*Diagnostic and Statistical Manual of
    Mental Disorders*, 12
Dialectical behavior therapy (DBT),
    118–120
Diaphragmatic breathing exercises,
    184–185
Disability, 233
Distractibility
    in depressive states, 19
    in manic and hypomanic states, 14
Distress tolerance skills, 119
Divorcing your partner, 229, 277–280.
    See also Relationship with your
    partner
Doctors
    collaboration between the doctors
        involved, 133–135
    depressive episode and, 242–248
    emergencies and, 224
    expectations of, 135–138
    family doctors, 91–93
    finding the right one, 87–93, 138

Doctors (*cont.*)
learning about bipolar disorder from, 168–169
manic or hypomanic episode and, 207, 209, 212–213
meeting with yourself, 128–133, 207, 209
psychiatrists and psychopharmacologists, 88–91
questions for, 169
suicide and, 251, 252
what to look for in, 89, 90
working with. *See* Team approach
Double depression, 40
Driving. *See also* Risk-taking behaviors
accidents and, 58–59
during a manic or hypomanic episode, 215–217
after a mood episode, 262
Drug use. *See* Substance abuse/use
Duration of mood episodes, 36–39. *See also* Course of bipolar disorder
Dysthymia, double depression and, 40

Early intervention plan
depressive episodes and, 242–248
mania and hypomania and, 209–213
when symptoms escalate too quickly for, 212–213, 244–248
Eating changes, in depressive states, 18
ECT (electroconvulsive therapy)
depressive episodes and, 248
overview, 111–112
side effects of, 112
Educating yourself and your partner about bipolar disorder, 167–171
Electroconvulsive therapy (ECT)
depressive episodes and, 248
overview, 111–112
side effects of, 112
Elevated mood, 10–11. *See also* Hypomania; Mania
Emergency
hospitalization and, 12, 58, 212, 213, 245, 249
meeting with doctors yourself and, 129
overview, 224
planning for, 129, 224, 255, 265
police and, 228, 252, 255
Emotion regulation skills, 119
Employers, telling about the condition and, 232–233

Exercise
early intervention and, 210–211, 242
taking care of yourself and, 276–277
Exhaustion, taking care of yourself and, 230
Exposure-based procedures, 117. *See also* Cognitive-behavioral therapy (CBT)
Extramarital affairs. *See* Infidelity

Family doctors, 91–93. *See also* Doctors
Family members with bipolar disorder, 77–80. *See also* Genetic factors in bipolar disorder
Family support groups, 124
Family-focused therapy (FFT), 121–123
Fatigued feeling, 19
Fear
cognitive-behavioral therapy and, 117
overview, 3
taking care of yourself and, 228
FFT (family-focused therapy), 121–123
Financial issues
during depression, 261–262
during a manic or hypomanic episode, 14–15, 214–215
after a mood episode, 261–262
Forms/worksheets/checklists
Mood Disorder Checklist, 80, 81, 82
Mood Disorders in Relatives form, 79
Mood Monitoring form, 178–180
Mood Rating Scale, 172–176
My Partner's Early Warning Signs of Depression form, 239
My Partner's Early Warning Signs of Mania form, 206
Negative Consequences of Manic/ Hypomanic Moods checklist, 163
Frequency of mood episodes, 33–36. *See also* Course of bipolar disorder
Full recovery between episodes, 39–40

Gender, course of bipolar disorder and, 50–54
Generalized anxiety disorder, 55
Genetic factors in bipolar disorder
age at the start of illness and, 50
children of people with bipolar disorder and, 4
the decision to have children and, 3–4, 52–53, 265–266
denial of the diagnosis and, 77–80

encouraging your partner to explore, 77–80
fear associated with, 3–4
Geodon, 102. *See also* Atypical antipsychotics; Medication
Goal setting, 242
Grandiose delusions, 26–27, 58, 221–222
Grandiosity
in manic and hypomanic states, 13
overview, 221–222
Gregariousness, 15
Group therapy
dialectical behavior therapy and, 118–120
overview, 124
Guilt
children of people with bipolar disorder and, 4
in depressive states, 19
genetic factors in bipolar disorder and, 4
taking care of yourself and, 227

Hallucinations. *See also* Psychotic features
atypical antipsychotics and, 101
depressive episodes and, 252–253
manic episodes and, 252–253
in manic versus hypomanic episodes, 12
overview, 222–225
safety and, 220–225
schizoaffective disorder and, 27
schizophrenia and, 26–27
Helplessness
helping your partner too much and, 140–142
overview, 3
taking care of yourself and, 257–258
Hopelessness
in depressive states, 20
taking care of yourself and, 230
Hormone levels
in bipolar women, 51–54
symptoms of that mimic those of bipolar disorder, 48
Hospitalization
benefits of, 249
depressive episodes and, 245
involuntary, 252
mania and, 212, 213
in manic versus hypomanic episodes, 12
overview, 213

planning ahead for, 213, 248, 252, 254
suicide and, 58
Hurtful things your spouse says to you, 228, 269–270
Hyperthyroidism, symptoms of that mimic those of bipolar disorder, 48
Hypomania
behavioral contract and, 225–226
benefits of bipolar disorder and, 59–60
changes in mood during, 10–11
cognitive-behavioral therapy and, 116
compared to mania, 12–17
consequences of, 200–201
cyclothymic disorder and, 22–23
early intervention plan and, 209–212
early warning signs of, 201–205
episodes of, 12–17
helping your partner deal with, 199–234
misdiagnosis of major depressive disorder and, 24–26
missing when on medication, 15, 59–60, 161–164
"Mood Disorder Checklist" and, 80–82
pleasantness of, 12–13
safety during, 213–225
seasonal patterns of, 44–45
symptoms of, 13–17
taking care of yourself and, 227–230
Hypothyroidism, 48

Identity, denial of the diagnosis and, 68–69
Impulsive behavior
accidents and, 58–59
borderline personality disorder and, 28
in manic and hypomanic states, 14–15
Indecisiveness, 19
Inertia loss, 18
Infidelity
consequences of, 218–219
dealing with after the mood episode has ended, 262–263
during a manic or hypomanic episode, 15, 218–219
Interest, loss of, 18
Internet resources. *See also* Resources
denial of the diagnosis and, 65
learning about bipolar disorder from, 170
list of, 284–287

Interpersonal and social rhythm therapy (IPSRT), 120–121
Interpersonal conflicts, 193–198
Interpersonal effectiveness skills, 119
Intervention planning, early
  depressive episodes and, 242–248
  mania and hypomania and, 209–213
  when symptoms escalate too quickly for, 212–213, 244–248
Intimacy, relationship with your partner, 266–267
IPSRT (interpersonal and social rhythm therapy), 120–121
Irritable mood, 10–11. *See also* Hypomania; Mania

Judgment impairment
  accidents and, 58–59
  alcohol use and, 188, 217
  cognitive-behavioral therapy and, 116
  depressive episodes and, 243, 252
  mania and hypomania and, 211, 213–214, 218, 219–220

Kindling theory, 35
Klonopin, 111. *See also* Benzodiazepines; Medication

Lamictal, 100–101. *See also* Anticonvulsants; Medication; Mood stabilizers
Leadership, as a benefit of bipolar disorder, 59–60
Learning about bipolar disorder, 167–171
Leaving your relationship, 227–280, 229. *See also* Relationship with your partner
Length of mood episodes, 36–39. *See also* Course of bipolar disorder
Lexapro, 107. *See also* Antidepressants; Medication
Libido changes
  in depression, 18, 175
  in manic and hypomanic states, 15, 218–219
  medication and, 108
  relationship with your partner and, 266–267
  taking care of yourself and, 258–259
Librium, 111. *See also* Benzodiazepines; Medication
Life events, stressful
  manic or hypomanic episode and, 211

smaller stressors, 46–47
  as a trigger for mood episodes, 45–47
Lifestyle changes, 166–167. *See also* Preventing mood episodes
Light therapy, 44, 113
Lithium, 96–98. *See also* Medication; Mood stabilizers
Loneliness, 228–229, 257
Loss of interest, 18

Major depressive disorder
  compared to bipolar disorder, 24–26
  diagnosis and, 21–22
  misdiagnosis of, 24–26
  women and bipolar and, 53
Mania
  behavioral contract and, 225–226
  benefits of bipolar disorder and, 59–60
  changes in mood during, 10–11
  cognitive-behavioral therapy and, 116
  compared to hypomania, 12–17
  consequences of, 200–201
  early intervention plan and, 209–212
  early warning signs of, 201–205
  episodes of, 12–17
  helping your partner deal with, 199–234
  misdiagnosis of major depressive disorder and, 24–26
  missing when on medication, 15, 59–60, 161–164
  "Mood Disorder Checklist" and, 80–82
  postpartum period and, 51–52
  safety during, 213–225
  seasonal patterns of, 44–45
  symptoms of, 13–17
  taking care of yourself and, 227–230
Manic–depression "switch"
  antidepressants and, 106
  overview, 37
  substance use and, 47
Medical conditions, 48
Medication. *See also* Medication compliance; *specific medications*; Treatment options
  ADHD and, 193
  alcohol use and, 191
  anticonvulsants, 98–101
  antidepressants, 106–109
  atypical antipsychotics, 101–106
  benefits of bipolar disorder and, 59–60
  benzodiazepines, 110–111

breakthrough episodes and, 34
compliance with, 145–164
decreasing the frequency of mood
    episodes and, 33–34
denial of the diagnosis and, 65–67, 83
diagnosis and, 21–22
duration of mood episodes and, 37
early warning sights of a manic
    episode and, 201, 212, 218–219
early warning signs of a depressive
    episode and, 245, 246, 248
encouraging your partner to accept,
    65–67, 83, 147–150, 151–152,
    157–160, 162–164
fears regarding, 65–67
finding the right doctor and, 87–93,
    92–93
forgetting to take, 155–156
learning about to help your partner,
    93–111
minimization of the problem and, 83
missing the highs when using, 16,
    59–60, 161–164
mood stabilizers, 96–101
not liking the idea of taking, 147–150
overmedicating and, 157
during pregnancy, 52–53
psychotic features and, 253
rapid cycling and, 51
reasons people may stop taking, 146
refusing to take, 65–67, 268–269
relationships and, 41
resistance to, 93–94
side effects of, 57, 94, 97, 99–100,
    100–101, 101, 102, 104–106,
    107–108, 111, 157–161
skills-oriented treatment and, 122
stopping, 93–94
trying several to find what works,
    94–95, 103
typical antipsychotics, 104–106
Medication compliance. See also
    Medication
feeling that medication isn't working
    and, 153–155
forgetting to take medication,
    155–156
missing the up periods and, 161–164
not liking the idea of taking
    medication, 147–150
overview, 145–146
side effects and, 157–161
when your partner is feeling better,
    150–153

Meditation practices
    dealing with recurrence and, 36
    dialectical behavior therapy and, 119
    taking care of yourself and, 142–143
Menopause, 53
Menstrual cycle
    PMS, 51–52
    women and bipolar and, 53
Metabolic syndrome
    atypical antipsychotics and, 102, 103
    cardiovascular disease and, 56–57
    suicide and, 58
    typical antipsychotics and, 104–106
Mindfulness
    dealing with recurrence and, 35–36
    dialectical behavior therapy and, 119
    taking care of yourself and, 142–143
Minimization of the problem. See also
        Denial of the diagnosis
    forgetting to take medication and, 155
    overview, 83–84
    self-help books and, 169
Mixed episodes
    age at the start of illness and, 50
    duration of, 37
    misdiagnosis of major depressive
        disorder and, 24–26
    overview, 20–21
    symptoms of, 20–21
Monamine oxidase inhibitor (MAOI)
        antidepressants, 107. See also
        Antidepressants; Medication
Money issues. See Financial issues
Monitoring moods. See Mood monitoring
Mood charting. See also Mood
        monitoring
    feeling that medication isn't working
        and, 153–154
    identifying precipitants of mood
        changes while, 178–179
    overview, 178–180
    preventing mood episodes by,
        179–180
Mood Disorder Checklist
    complete, 81
    overview, 80, 82
Mood Disorders in Relatives form, 79
Mood episodes. See also Preventing
        mood episodes
    in between, 39–42
    depressive episodes, 17–20
    duration of, 36–39
    frequency of, 34–35
    manic and hypomanic episodes, 12–17

medical treatments for, 93–111, 94–95, 103
mixed episodes, 20–21
overview, 12
preventing, 165–198
reacting to your partner during, 38
recovering after, 261–265
skills oriented therapies for, 114–124
Mood fluctuations, normal, 180–181
Mood monitoring. *See also* Mood charting
charting moods and, 178–180
Mood Rating Scale, 172–176
overview, 171–181
Mood Monitoring form
complete, 179
overview, 178–180
Mood Rating Scale
complete, 174–175
overview, 172–176
Mood stabilizers. *See also* Medication
antidepressants and, 106, 245
overview, 96–101
Mood Triggers inventory, 176–178, 177
Mortality risks, 56–59
Moving
desire to return to an earlier setting and, 75–76
preventing mood episodes and, 187
as a trigger for mood episodes, 45–46
Muscle relaxation, 184–185
My Partner's Early Warning Signs of Depression form, 239
My Partner's Early Warning Signs of Mania form, 206

Negative Consequences of Manic/ Hypomanic Moods checklist, 163
Negative thoughts, 116, 238, 246
Normal mood fluctuations, 180–181

Obesity
cardiovascular disease and, 56–57
suicide and, 58
Obsessive–compulsive disorder, 55
Olfactory hallucinations, 222–225. *See also* Hallucinations
Online resources. *See also* Resources
denial of the diagnosis and, 65
learning about bipolar disorder from, 170
support groups and, 171
Organizations, resources for, 287–291

Overmedication, 157. *See also* Medication
Overprotectiveness of your partner, 141. *See also* Taking care of yourself

Panic disorder, 55
Paranoid delusions, 27, 214
Paranoid thoughts
borderline personality disorder and, 28
mania and, 17, 27, 28, 202, 204, 221–222
overview, 221–222
Parenting
during a manic episode, 219–220
after a mood episode, 263–264
Partial recovery between episodes, 39–40
Paxil, 106, 107. *See also* Antidepressants; Medication
Personality
characteristics often seen in partners of people with bipolar disorder, 8
denial of the diagnosis and, 68–69
distinguishing between the disorder and one's "self," 69, 70
overview, 28–29
Personality disorders, 28, 55
Pessimism, 116
Phobias
cognitive-behavioral therapy and, 117
overview, 55
Phototherapy
early intervention plan for, 209–210, 243
overview, 44, 113
Physical activity
early intervention plan for, 210–211, 242
taking care of yourself and, 276–277
Planning, dealing with recurrence and, 36
Pleasant events, 242–243
PMS, 51–52
Postpartum period, 52–53
Posttraumatic stress disorder, 55
Premenstrual syndrome (PMS), 51–52
Present life, living in
dealing with recurrence and, 35–36
taking care of yourself and, 142–143
Pressured speech, 16
Preventing mood episodes. *See also* Lifestyle changes; Risk factors; Triggers of mood episodes; Warning signs of mood episodes

alcohol use and, 188–193
behavioral contract and, 225–226
identifying early warning signs and, 201–205, 205–209, 209–212, 225–226, 237–241, 242–248, 248–253
learning about bipolar disorder and, 167–171
medication and, 201, 212, 218–219, 245, 246, 248
mood monitoring and, 171–181
overview, 165–167
problem solving and, 243
resolving interpersonal conflicts and, 193–198
routines and, 185–187
skills oriented therapies and, 114–124
sleep hygiene and, 181–185
triggers of mood episodes and, 171–181
Privacy, meeting with doctors yourself and, 130–131
Problem solving, 117
Productivity, 14, 15
Promiscuity, 218–219
Prozac, 107. *See also* Antidepressants; Medication
Psychiatric hospitalization. *See* Hospitalization
Psychiatrists, 88–91. *See also* Doctors
Psychoeducation, 167–171
Psychopharmacologists, 88–91. *See also* Doctors
Psychotic features. *See also* Delusions; Hallucinations
accidents and, 58–59
atypical antipsychotics and, 101
depressive episodes and, 252–253
manic episodes and, 220–225
in manic versus hypomanic episodes, 12
mortality rates and, 58–59
safety and, 220–225
schizoaffective disorder and, 27
schizophrenia and, 26–27

Racing thoughts, 16
Rage, during mania and hypomania, 11
Rapid transcranial magnetic stimulation (rTMS), 112
Rapid cycling
age at the start of illness and, 50
antidepressants and causing, 47
definition of, 21

gender and, 50–51
women and bipolar and, 53
Recovery between episodes
complete, 50, 67
deteriorating course, 41–42
overview, 39–40
partial, 50, 67
reconnecting with others and, 41
Recurrence, 35–36
Rejection of the diagnosis. *See* Denial of the diagnosis
Relationship with your partner. *See also* Relationships with others; Taking care of yourself
caretaker role, 267–268
challenges to, 265–270
denial and, 61–62
during a depressive episode, 236
leaving or ending, 229, 277–280
during a manic or hypomanic episodes, 229
meeting with doctors yourself and, 132
after a mood episode, 261–265
taking care of, 260–281
Relationships with others. *See also* Relationship with your partner
conflict resolution and, 193–198
depressive episodes and, 236, 243
interpersonal and social rhythm therapy and, 120–121
reconnecting during remission and, 41
telling others about the condition and, 231–234
Relaxation exercises, 184–185
Relocation. *See* Moving
Remission, reconnecting with others during, 41
Residential treatment programs
alcohol abuse/dependence and, 191
dual diagnosis and, 191, 193
leaving or ending your relationship and, 280
Resources
books to read, 283–284
cognitive-behavioral therapy and, 118
denial of the diagnosis and, 65
dialectical behavior therapy and, 120
family-focused therapy and, 123
Internet resources, 170, 284–287
interpersonal and social rhythm therapy and, 121
list of, 283–291

Resources (*cont.*)
  organizations, 287–291
  self-help books, 169–170
Restlessness, 15
Reverse diurnal variation, 44
Risk factors for mood episodes. *See also*
    Preventing mood episodes; Triggers
    of mood episodes
  list of, 168
  medication inconsistency as, 146, 168
  postpartum period as, 52–53
  premenstrual syndrome (PMS) as,
    51–52
Risk-taking behaviors
  accidents and, 58–59, 215–217
  alcohol use and, 188, 217–218
  borderline personality disorder and,
    28
  cognitive-behavioral therapy and, 116
  dialectical behavior therapy and, 119
  extramarital affairs, 15, 218–219
  in manic and hypomanic states,
    14–15, 213–224
  money and, 214–215
  safety and, 213–225
Routines, daily
  changes in as a trigger for mood
    episodes, 43–44
  cognitive-behavioral therapy and, 117
  decreasing the frequency of mood
    episodes and, 33
  early intervention plan and, 210, 243
  interpersonal and social rhythm
    therapy and, 120
  overview, 167, 185–187
  preventing mood episodes and,
    185–187
  sleep hygiene and, 182
  sleep–wake cycle disturbances and,
    42–43
  traveling and disruption of, 168, 185,
    186–187
rTMS (rapid transcranial magnetic
    stimulation), 112

Sadness, 227–228, 256–257. *See*
    Depression
Safety
  hospitalization and, 218
  during a depressive episode, 252
  during a manic or hypomanic episode,
    213–225
  suicide and, 252

Sample Contract for Suicide Prevention
    form, 254
Schedules, daily. *See also* Routines, daily
  cognitive-behavioral therapy and, 117
  interpersonal and social rhythm
    therapy and, 120
  preventing mood episodes and,
    185–187
  sleep hygiene and, 182
Scheduling worry time technique,
    184–185
Schizoaffective disorder, 27
Schizophrenia, 26–27, 54–55
Seasonal affective disorder, 23, 44
Seasonal patterns, as a trigger for mood
    episodes, 44–45
Second opinions, denial of the diagnosis
    and, 76–77
Self-absorption, depressive episodes
    and, 236
Self-confidence, 13
Self-hatred, 19
Self-help books, 169–170
Self-help groups
  alcohol use and, 191, 192
  overview, 124, 171
Self-help strategies, 41
Self-importance, in manic and
    hypomanic states, 13
Seroquel, 102. *See also* Atypical
    antipsychotics; Medication
Sex drive
  infidelity, 15, 218–219, 262–263
  in manic and hypomanic states, 15,
    218–219
  relationship with your partner and,
    266–267
  taking care of yourself and, 258–259
Shame, denial of the diagnosis and, 68
"Shock therapy," 111–112
Side effects of medication. *See*
    Medication
Skills-oriented treatments, 114–124
Sleep deprivation treatment, 114
Sleep disturbances
  course of bipolar disorder and, 42–43
  in depressive states, 18
  helping your partner with, 181–185
  interpersonal and social rhythm
    therapy and, 121
  in manic and hypomanic states, 14
  as a trigger for mood episodes, 42–43
Sleep hygiene, 181–185

Sleep–wake cycle, 42–43
Sociability, 15
Social anxiety disorder, 55
Social stimulation
  early intervention plan and, 210
  interpersonal and social rhythm
    therapy, 120–121
  preventing mood episodes and, 186
  taking care of yourself and, 276–277
Spectrum of bipolar disorders, 10
Speech, pressured, 16
Spending issues. *See* Financial issues
SSNRIs, 107. *See also* Antidepressants;
  Medication
SSRIs, 107. *See also* Antidepressants;
  Medication
Steps to wellness, list of, 143–144
Steroids, as a trigger for mood episodes,
  48–49
Stress management skills
  cognitive-behavioral therapy and, 117
  skills-oriented treatment and, 122
Stressful life events
  smaller stressors, 46–47
  as a trigger for mood episodes, 45–46,
    211
Substance abuse
  during depressive episodes, 38, 49,
    248–249
  during mania and hypomania,
    213–214
  treatment for, 188–193, 213
Substance abuse/use
  abuse versus dependence, 192
  duration of mood episodes and, 38
  during mania and hypomania, 22
  overview, 29–30, 55
  preventing mood episodes and,
    188–193
  suicide and, 57–58
  as a trigger for mood episodes, 47–49
Suicidal thoughts or behaviors
  borderline personality disorder and,
    28
  dealing with after the mood episode
    has ended, 264–265
  depressive episodes and, 19, 249–252
  dialectical behavior therapy and, 119
  hospitalization and, 58, 251–252, 254
  lithium and, 96
  manic or hypomanic episodes and,
    220
  mixed episodes and, 21, 220, 224

  mortality rates and, 57–58
  overview, 57–58
  safety and, 252
  Sample Contract for Suicide
    Prevention form, 254
  taking care of yourself and, 255
  warning signs of, 250–252
  what you should do when your
    partner has, 249–252
Sun exposure, 209–210. *See also*
  Phototherapy
  early intervention plan for depressive
    episodes, 243
  early intervention plan for manic and
    hypomanic episodes and, 209–210
  hypomanic episodes and, 209–210
Support for you, 272–277. *See also*
  Taking care of yourself
Support groups, 124, 171
"Switch," manic–depression
  antidepressants and, 106
  overview, 37
  substance use and, 47
Symbyax, 108. *See also* Antidepressants;
  Medication
Symptoms. *See also* Warning signs of
  mood episodes
  of depressive states, 17–20
  as early warning signs of manic or
    hypomanic episodes, 201–205
  as early warning signs of of a
    depressive episode, 237–241
  increasing of, 212–213
  of manic or hypomanic states, 13–17
  of mixed states, 20–21
  Mood Rating Scale, 172–176
  severity of, 171–172, 181–182
  type I and type II bipolar disorder
    and, 21–22

Tactile hallucinations, 222–225. *See
  also* Hallucinations
Taking care of yourself. *See also*
  Relationship with your partner
  caretaker role and, 267–268
  coping skills and, 142–143
  expectations of yourself and, 138–140
  finding support, 272–277
  helping too much and, 139, 140–142,
    267–268
  identifying your needs and, 270–272
  leaving or ending your relationship
    and, 229, 277–280

Taking care of yourself (*cont.*)
    after a mood episode, 261–265
    overview, 127–128, 260–281
    supporting yourself and, 276–277
    during your partner's depressive
        episodes, 253–259
    during your partner's manic or
        hypomanic episodes, 227–230
Tardive dyskinesia, 105–106. *See also*
    Medication
Team approach. *See also* Doctors
    collaboration between the doctors
        involved, 133–135
    expectations of your partner's doctor,
        135–138
    expectations of yourself, 138–143
    helping too much and, 140–142
    meeting with doctors yourself,
        128–133
    overview, 125–128
    your role as a team member, 125–128,
        128–133
Telling others about the condition
    children and, 263–264
    coworkers, 233–234
    employers, 232–233
    friends, 231–232
    overview, 231–234
    relatives, 231–232
The Bipolar Disorder Survival Guide
    (Miklowitz), 65
Therapy
    alcohol use and, 191
    cognitive-behavioral therapy (CBT),
        115–118
    comparison of, 123
    consistency and, 152
    denial of the diagnosis and, 137
    dialectical behavior therapy (DBT),
        118–120
    expectations of your partner's
        therapist and, 137
    family-focused therapy (FFT),
        121–123
    goals of, 122
    interpersonal and social rhythm
        therapy (IPSRT), 120–121
    self-help and support groups, 124
    what you and your partner can expect
        from, 114–124
Thyroid
    augmentation, 114
    lithium and, 98

symptoms of that mimic those of
        bipolar disorder, 48
Tired, feeling, 19
Tranxene, 111. *See also* Benzodiazepines;
    Medication
Travelling
    preventing mood episodes and,
        186–187
    triggers of mood episodes and, 43–44
Treatment. *See also* Medication;
        Treatment, learning about;
        Treatment seeking
    alcohol use and, 191
    benefits of bipolar disorder and,
        59–60
    consistency and, 152
    course of bipolar disorder and, 32
    decreasing the frequency of mood
        episodes and, 33–34
    early intervention plan and, 209–212,
        209–213, 242–248, 244–248
    medical options other than
        medication, 111–114
    partner's refusal of, 268–269
    skills oriented therapies, 114–124
    substance use and, 49
    for your children, 263–264
Treatment, learning about. *See also*
        Treatment; Treatment seeking
    medication and, 93–111
    other medical options, 111–114
    overview, 86–87
    the right doctor and, 87–93
    self-help and support groups, 124
    skills oriented therapies, 114–124
Treatment seeking. *See also* Treatment;
        Treatment, learning about
    acceptance of the diagnosis and, 63
    denial of the diagnosis and, 69–84
    finding the right doctor, 87–93, 138
    helping your partner take that step,
        69–84
    misdiagnosis of major depressive
        disorder and, 24
Tricyclic antidepressants, 107. *See also*
    Antidepressants; Medication
Triggers of mood episodes. *See also*
        Preventing mood episodes; Risk
        factors for mood episodes
    anxiety as, 46–47, 117, 168, 176–178,
        180
    changes in routine as, 43–44
    course of bipolar disorder and, 42–49

decreasing the frequency of mood
    episodes and, 33, 35
identifying, 171–181
interpersonal conflict, 193–198
mania and hypomania and, 201, 211
medical conditions as, 48
mood monitoring and, 171–181
seasonal patterns and, 44–45
skills-oriented treatments and, 122
sleep–wake cycle disturbances and,
    42–43, 181–185
stressful life events as, 45–47
substance abuse and, 47–49
12-step programs, 191, 192
Type I bipolar disorder
    diagnosis of, 21–22
    duration of mood episodes and, 37
    overview, 55
    risk of bipolar II disorder turning into,
        55–56
Type II bipolar disorder
    diagnosis of, 21–22
    duration of mood episodes and, 37
    overview, 55–56
    risk of turning into bipolar I disorder,
        55–56
Typical antipsychotics, 104–106. See
    also Medication

Ultimatitums, giving to your partner
    verbal abuse and, 269–270
Ultimatums, giving to your partner
    regarding medication compliance,
        149–150
Uncertainty about the future, 31–32.
    See also Course of bipolar disorder
Unipolar depression, 21–22
Unpredictable nature of bipolar
    disorder, 31–32. See also Course of
    bipolar disorder

Vacations
    preventing mood episodes and,
        186–187
    triggers of mood episodes and, 43–44

Vagus nerve stimulation (VNS), 113
Valium, 111. See also Benzodiazepines;
    Medication
Verbal abuse by your partner, 228,
    269–270
Visual hallucinations, 222–225. See also
    Hallucinations
Vitamin B deficiencies, 48
VNS (vagus nerve stimulation), 113

Warning signs of mood episodes. See
    also Preventing mood episodes;
    Symptoms
    behavioral contract and, 225–226
    decreasing the frequency of mood
        episodes and, 33
    depressive episodes and, 237–241,
        248–253
    early intervention plan and, 209–212,
        242–248
    mania and hypomania and, 201–205
    recognizing in your partner, 127
    skills-oriented treatment and, 122
    what you can do when you notice,
        205–209, 248–253
Websites. See Internet resources
Wellbutrin, 106, 107. See also
    Antidepressants; Medication
Work, telling about the condition and,
    232–233
Worksheets. See Forms/worksheets/
    checklists
Worry, 184–185, 255. See also Anxiety
    overview, 3
Worthlessness, feelings of, 19

Xanax, 111. See also Benzodiazepines;
    Medication

Zoloft, 107. See also Antidepressants;
    Medication
Zyprexa, 101–102. See also Atypical
    antipsychotics; Medication

About the Author

Cynthia G. Last, PhD, is a clinical psychologist in private practice in Boca Raton, Florida. She has served on the faculties of the University of Pittsburgh School of Medicine and Nova Southeastern University, and is internationally known for her research on the diagnosis and treatment of psychological disorders. The author or editor of 13 books, Dr. Last has been widely quoted and interviewed in the media. She lives with her husband of more than 20 years, Barry M. Rubin.